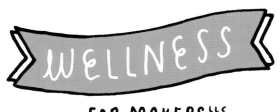

FOR MAKERS LLC

WELLNESS
FOR
MAKERS

a Movement Guide for Artists

MISSY GRAFF BALLONE

Images by Eye Spy Photography

Illustrations by Julianna Brazill

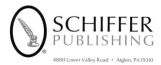

SCHIFFER
PUBLISHING

4880 Lower Valley Road • Atglen, PA 19310

Other Schiffer Books on
Related Subjects:

Artists Write to Work, Kate Kramer,
ISBN 978-0-7643-5649-0

Branding + Interior Design, Kim Kuhteubl,
ISBN 978-0-7643-5129-7

Master Your Craft, Tien Chiu,
ISBN 978-0-7643-5145-7

Cover and interior design by Ashley Millhouse
Type set in Agenda

ISBN: 978-0-7643-6321-4
Printed in India

Published by Schiffer Publishing, Ltd.
4880 Lower Valley Road
Atglen, PA 19310
Phone: (610) 593-1777; Fax: (610) 593-2002
Email: Info@schifferbooks.com
Web: www.schifferbooks.com

For our complete selection of fine books on this and related subjects, please visit
our website at www.schifferbooks.com. You may also write for a free catalog.

Schiffer Publishing's titles are available at special discounts for bulk purchases for
sales promotions or premiums. Special editions, including personalized covers,
corporate imprints, and excerpts, can be created in large quantities for special
needs. For more information, contact the publisher.

We are always looking for people to write books on new and related subjects. If
you have an idea for a book, please contact us at proposals@schifferbooks.com.

A stitch in time
may save nine.

—Anonymous, ca. 1733[1]

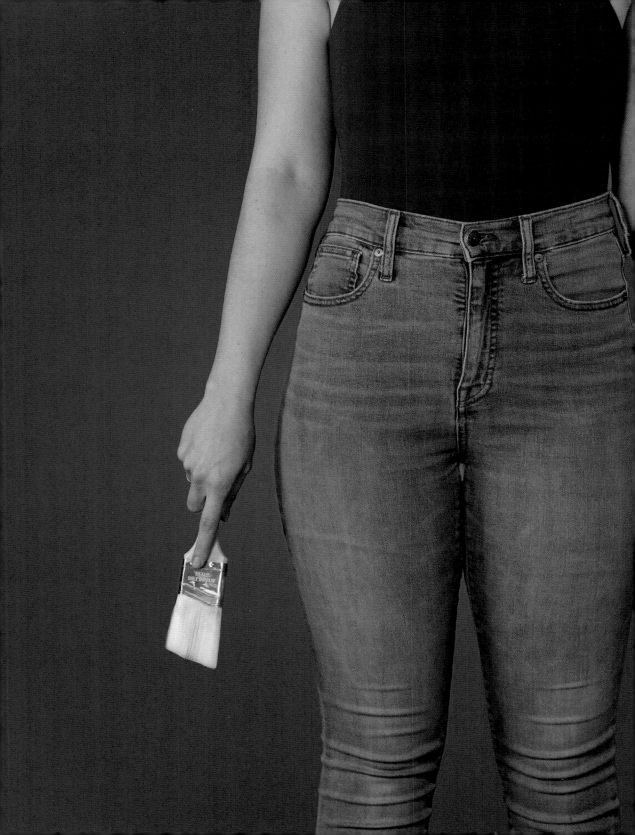

Table of Contents

Author's Note

The information in this book is solely for informational purposes and is not intended to diagnose, treat, cure, or prevent disease or to provide medical advice. Please consult a licensed physician or other healthcare professional for your specific healthcare and medical needs or concerns. The content in this book is not intended to be a substitute for professional medical advice, diagnosis, or treatments. It is your responsibility to seek the advice of a licensed physician or other qualified healthcare provider with any question you may have regarding a medical condition and before undertaking any new healthcare regimen. Never disregard professional medical advice or delay in seeking it because of something you have learned in this book.

Please note that all movement programs pose inherent risk of bodily injury. Participation in any of the techniques or strategies described in this book is therefore done at your own risk. The author and publisher disclaim liability for any injuries or damages to anyone as a result of following the information, exercises, and movements in this book. The information in this book is accurate to the best of the author's knowledge; however, we are not responsible for any damages caused by errors, omissions, or mistakes in this book.

All product recommendations are provided for your convenience only, and use of these products is done at your own risk. We make no representations or warranties of any kind, express or implied, as to the information or recommended products.

The text and products pictured in this book are from the collection of the author of this book, its publisher, or various private collectors. This book is not sponsored, endorsed, or otherwise affiliated with any of the companies whose products are represented herein. This book is derived from the author's independent research.

INTRODUCTION

My passion for learning about the human body began when I injured my knee and tore my ACL during a gymnastics practice in 2005. The ACL is one of the key ligaments that stabilizes the knee joint, and I had to undergo reconstructive surgery along with months of physical therapy to recover. During my physical therapy sessions, I worked hard to build strength, and each week I gained more mobility. I also began to learn about the interior structures of the body, injury, and how we heal.

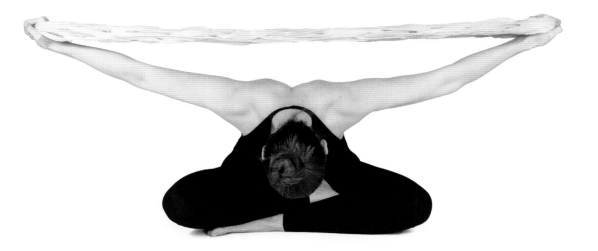

This experience taught me how resilient the body is. Resilience is the body's ability to recover from injury and spring back into shape: elasticity! Elasticity also refers to the ability of our soft tissues to resume their original shapes after being stretched, compressed, or massaged. The resilience of your tissues supports mobility by allowing you to safely exercise your body's range of motion. I was also starting to understand what it meant to have more kinesthetic awareness, and it felt empowering! Soon after my physical therapy sessions ended, I began practicing yoga asana to maintain strength and flexibility. It was around this time that I spent a few months traveling throughout California and developed an interest in massage therapy. I loved the idea of having a job I could be passionate about while I worked my way through art school, so I enrolled in a program to become a licensed massage therapist.

A few years later, while I was working toward my master of fine arts, a professor asked me why I felt that it's important to mention that I'm a massage therapist in my introductions. That part of my education was important to me, and I wanted both worlds to intersect. From that point on, my artwork became heavily influenced by my tactile understanding of the body.

The idea for Wellness for Makers® was not far behind. While I was at Peter's Valley School of Craft in 2014, I was having a conversation with a group of craftsmen about the pain that artists often experience as a result of their studio practices. One member of the group suggested that we should all accept that we will eventually develop a repetitive strain injury (arthritis or carpal tunnel syndrome).

The more conversations I had about these issues, the more I saw a need for wellness education in the arts. I felt a strong sense of responsibility to use my background in massage therapy and wellness to educate other artists about how to create more-healthful studio habits. I have been a massage therapist since 2007. In order to maintain my license and stay up to date with the most relevant information about the body and movement, I complete continuing education credits each year. When I realized that wellness education was lacking in the arts, I decided to focus my continued studies on learning accessible self-care and movement techniques that I could bring back to the artist studio. As my passion for movement, alignment, and posture grew, I also completed over 800 hours of alignment-based yoga teacher training, advanced my studies in kinesiology taping methods, self-massage techniques, and more.

I believe that information about the body and movement should be more accessible to artists everywhere. You should not have to complete the number of programs I have or will in order to develop more awareness in your body. My goal in all of this research and continued study has been to transform the information that I've learned and break it down into digestible ideas for you to try in your own studio practice.

When you learn to move well, your body has the ability to mend itself one thread at a time. *Wellness for Makers: A Movement Guide for Artists* will teach you how to alleviate pain and strain while working in the studio through active and passive stretching, strengthening, and massage techniques that are easy to incorporate into your daily routine.

The content in this book is from my unique perspective and training up to this point. I will also share examples from my personal research and experience to offer you invitations and considerations. I will explain common misalignments in the artist studio to help you understand what's happening in your own body. I will deconstruct posture positions and teach you how to create strength through your movement patterns. This book is not a quick-fix guide. The techniques take time, effort, and consistency to practice. Some movements may help you experience immediate temporary relief, while others will empower you to engage with your creative vision more fully over time.

Moving your body should be a joy, not a chore.

- Erwan Le Corre, Creator of Movnat.

The Practice of Natural Movement: Reclaim Power, Health, and Freedom

CHAPTER 1 WHY WE MOVE

I believe you will be much more likely to create a practice that lasts if you redefine what movement means to you. Your body is always moving in one way or another. You are breathing, your beautiful heart is beating, and your incredible mind is working. Even when you are sitting still, your body is dynamically supporting you.

Movement is so much more than just exercise. Your body needs a variety of movements in order to create and maintain longevity, build strength and stability, and develop mobility.[1] However, because we live sedentary lifestyles, we need to find ways to incorporate significantly more movement back into our lives. It's no secret that the act of sitting for long periods of time comes with its own health risks.[2] The good news is that mixing up the time you spend standing or sitting in one position and actively engaging with a more diverse range of movements is enough to create positive change in your body.[3]

Have you ever heard the phrase "If you don't move it, you lose it!"? It means that if you don't use a particular part of your body for a specific movement, your body will think you no longer need access to that movement. If you rarely lift your arms over your head, for example, your body is going to limit your access to that motion and offer you stability instead by laying down extra connective tissue around your shoulder. Over time, it will become harder and harder to access an unused movement. This is how your body responds to your default movement patterns in order to conserve energy.[4]

Your body is always adapting based on the movements that you actually engage with. Incorporating more variety into your everyday movements will improve how you feel. Throughout the chapters in this book, I will invite you to get up and stretch, try a new technique, stand up and walk around, or change position. At the end of each chapter, you will be invited to reflect on your experiences with movement journal prompts to fill in. My goal is to remind you to notice your movement patterns as much as possible. Checking in with your body more often you will teach you how to build more kinesthetic awareness. Gaining more awareness is the first step to creating lasting change in your body. Remember that movement is a skill we learn and develop over time. Every moment is an opportunity to improve!

CHAPTER 2 WHY WE MEND

I've been inspired to learn new mending techniques. The practice has created space for some interesting considerations in my own life. Mending is the action of repair. As artists, we often have no problem making time for repairing our favorite tools, mending clothing, or even transforming our process based on the materials we are using. So why are many makers reluctant to offer themselves the same amount of love, care, and protection?

We often know what we need to do in order to feel great in our body, yet we put ourselves on the back burner. What happens when you do that with a piece of clothing? If there is a hole in my jeans and I continue to wear them over and over again with the mindset that "I will get to fixing this later" it is inevitable that the hole in the garment will eventually get bigger and bigger until it is much harder to repair. It is the same in the body. If you ignore the pain signals your body sends you with the mindset that you will take a break or switch your task sometime in the future and then never get to it, what should we anticipate happening? When you ignore the signals your body provides you with, you put yourself at risk of injury. Yet somehow, we are still surprised when we get there. We end up blaming our bad hands, our age, our bad backs, etc. Why not notice the movement pattern that you have created, deconstruct it, and fabricate a new one?

 I have met too many artists who are willing to accept that they are likely to develop chronic pain and injury as a result of their studio practice.

Everyone can benefit from learning more about the body, the way we move, and the way we heal. What does the word "mending" mean to you? Creatives often think of repairing an old pair of jeans with thread to make the area stronger than it once was. Mending an item of clothing creates longevity in the garment. In return for your efforts, you are able to wear it again and again without disregarding it.

You have the same opportunity to create longevity and strength in your body! Our tissues repair themselves in nonlinear ways all the time. Moving well and moving more increases your body's capacity to mend itself.[1] Your body is the most valuable tool you have. It will be easier to create longevity if we care for ourselves along the way rather than waiting for an injury to strike and then doing something about it.

I have worked with thousands of makers, and I often hear "I have terrible posture" or "I'm just getting older." Have you ever said something like this to yourself? Change in the body is inevitable, and we are constantly creating change whether we are conscious of it or not. We have the opportunity to decide how we want to engage with that process. You can either blame your body for aches, strains, and headaches or become more aware of how your everyday movements are affecting how you feel. Developing a stronger sense of kinesthetic awareness will empower you to find the relief you deserve. The fact that you are reading this book shows that you are already taking steps to create lasting change. Yes, it takes effort, but the good news is that even the smallest shifts and micro movements can create positive change in the body.

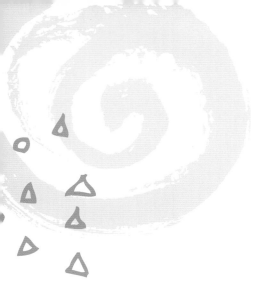

CHAPTER 3 FINDING NEUTRAL

My training as a massage therapist did not stop me from throwing my back out two years in a row during art school. Not only was I in pain, I also felt embarrassed for not knowing better. The second time, my chiropractor recommended that I re-evaluate not just the way I was moving in the studio, but also the way I was standing and sitting.

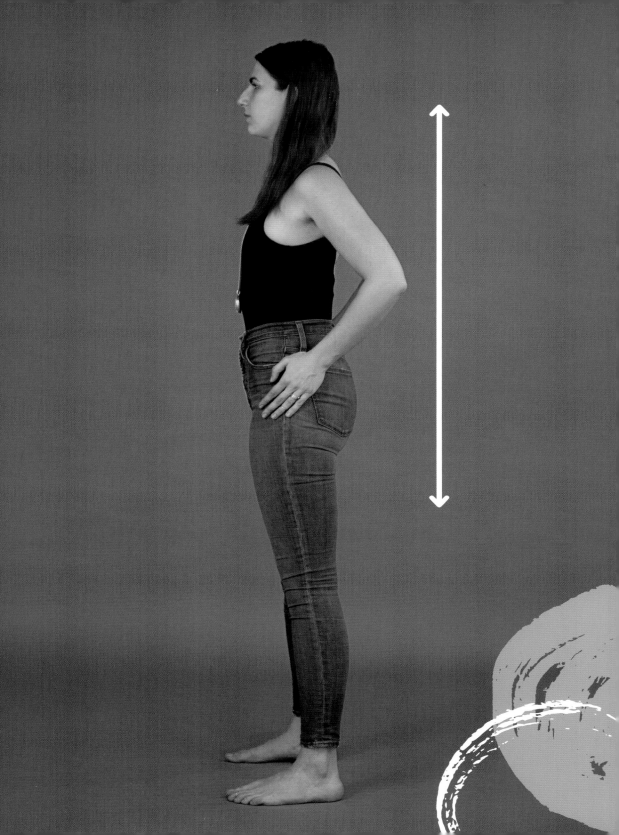

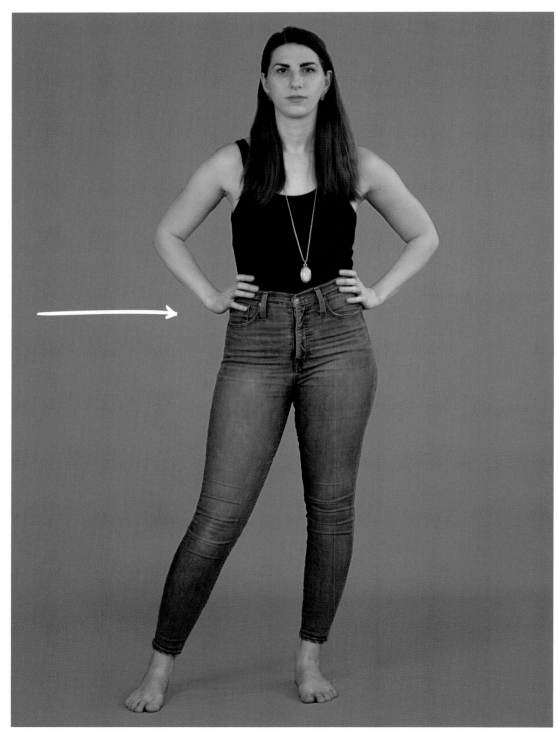

Leaning to one side

I was always uncomfortable while standing around for critiques because my default standing position involved shifting my weight to one side. I noticed that when I was in that position, the muscles on the left side of my back shortened and compressed and the muscles on my right side lengthened and overstretched. When you shift your weight to one side, it forces your pelvis to tilt out of neutral, which is fine temporarily but, when done repetitively, can cause issues.

What seemed like a harmless movement was creating unnecessary aches and pains throughout my body. What I didn't realize at the time was that I could make subtle adjustments in order to find relief. All of your muscles work together to control your movements, but when some muscles have to work extra hard because of the way you stand or sit, they can eventually become too fatigued to protect your body during everyday movements.

Anatomical neutral is a reference point for language about human anatomy and movement. If you've attended a yoga asana class, the posture is also called Tadasana. This is your home base when it comes to alignment. It is not to say that you should maintain this one position all day long or while working on particular tasks, but checking in with anatomical neutral allows you to learn how far away from it you come throughout the day.

It is important to develop movement patterns that distribute the loads of your studio practice evenly. As you learn what neutral looks and feels like in your body, you can use it as a reference for your other postures. Adjusting the alignment of your body to create more neutrality while you work can help you sit, stand, and move more effectively.[1]

My goal in teaching you about anatomical neutral is not to teach you how to maintain "perfect posture" all the time. It is unrealistic to stay in one position all day long. I consider anatomical neutral to be an excellent baseline to help you understand those movements.

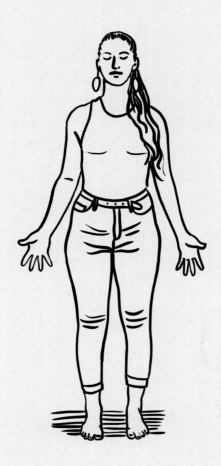

Proprioception vs. Kinesthesia: What's the Difference?

Proprioception and kinesthesia (also known as kinesthetic awareness) are two terms that are often misused interchangeably. They are not the same, but they do both relate to movement. Proprioception is the awareness of how your body is positioned in space, and includes your ability to balance. Proprioception is mostly subconscious and based on the angles and pressures of your joints at a specific point in time. Kinesthesia is the active awareness of your movements as they are happening. It is the sense you engage with as you develop a "feel" for a new technique. For example, when a jeweler is learning to texture a piece of metal with a chasing hammer, they might miss and hit their thumb by mistake. Kinesthesia is what detects the movement, if it was successful, and allows the maker to develop more control over time.[2]

Sitting vs. Standing

It's no secret that we are living in a time where our lifestyles are becoming more sedentary. Consider how many hours you sit throughout the day (working, driving, relaxing). Our bodies are designed to move. Studies have shown that sitting leads to, or is correlated with, a number of significant health risks, including chronic pain and disease.[3]

When you sit for extended periods of time, it is natural for your back to curve and round forward toward your work. This action causes unnecessary stress and uneven pressure on the spine, creating physically less space for the breath because the thoracic cavity is compressed and shortened. When you lengthen your spine, you can breathe more fully.

On its own, standing instead of sitting is not enough to counteract the health risks of being sedentary, and any form of prolonged inactivity creates risk, because our bodies are built to move.[4] Alternating between sitting and standing more often gives your joints and muscles a break from staying in any one static position for too long, and it encourages you to move more. Movement creates more circulation to support all of your biological functions. Sitting well can be a workout in itself when performed with intention. The issue is that if you weren't taught how to have good alignment while sitting, chances are your favorite standing posture is also unbalanced, leading to a different set of aches and pains.

Learning to sit and stand well might seem like a simple concept. However, if you look around at your studio mates, coworkers, classmates, and loved ones, you will likely notice that very few people actually stand and sit with a more neutral alignment. The good news is that you have the ability to develop stronger alignment in your standing and seated postures, find more opportunities to engage with movement, and gain more kinesthetic awareness.

Movement Break

Remember that movement means to change position. This means that a movement break doesn't have to be complicated or elaborate. Do what feels good to you. Move, bend, dance, or wiggle. Set a reminder to break up your sedentary position and switch shape every twenty minutes. Take a lap around the room, stretch, massage your hands, move from sitting to standing, or enjoy a glass of water. The more you listen to the signals of your body, the more positive results you will notice over time.

Standing Postures

In order to find neutral, it's helpful to check in with your own default positions. The natural curves of your spine help distribute force evenly, reduce pressure on your disks, and create space for your nerves to exit the spinal column and connect with the rest of your body. When you are standing farther away from anatomical neutral, specific areas of your body can become stressed or overloaded.

For example, hyperextension is when a joint, such as your knee, is pushed beyond the safe range of motion where your muscles can control its movement and guard it from injury. When a joint is in hyperextension, the ligaments around it act like brakes to create extra resistance to further movement in unsafe directions. Your ligaments are much less pliable than your muscles, which is good because it means they can absorb a lot of force even if it happens quickly. It also means that if you're not careful, you can easily develop a habit of using the strength of your ligaments instead of your muscles for a specific posture or action. Hyperextension in the knees often happens when the pelvis is misaligned too far in one direction. When the knee is "locked," it can feel very stable, but it can cause unnecessary strain over time. Maintaining a micro bend in your knees is an easy way to create muscle engagement and help keep them safe.

Look at the following images. Which standing postures do you find yourself in most throughout the day? We often think that we are more upright than we actually are. It can be helpful to have a mirror in your studio space to get a more accurate picture of how you stand, sit, and bend while you're making. Becoming aware of the postures you're in the most can help you see how far in and out of neutral you move throughout the day.

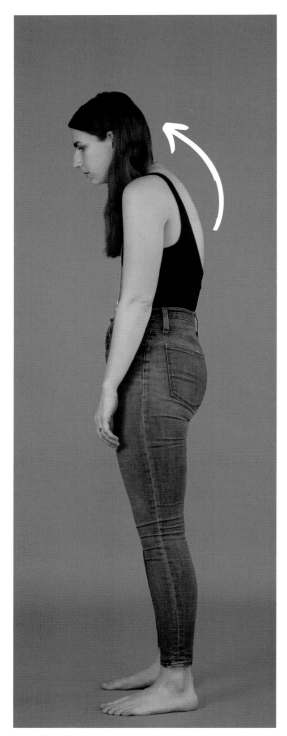

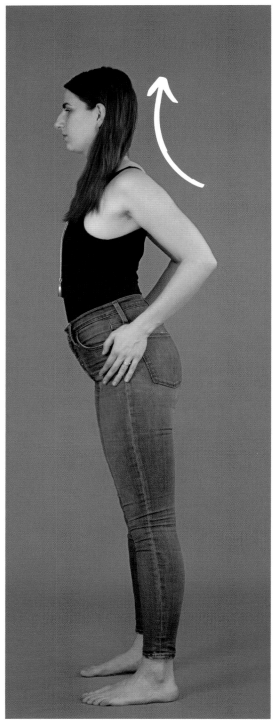

Hunched over

Exaggerated anterior tilt of the pelvis.
A common overcorrection.

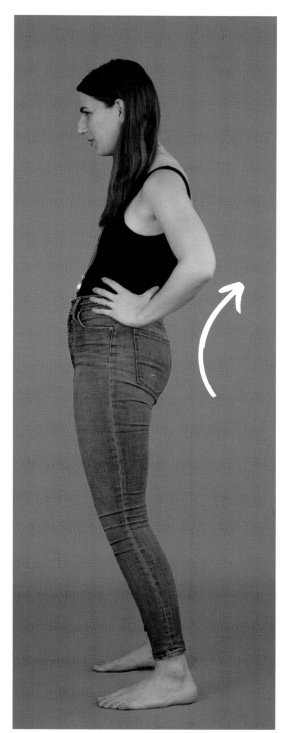

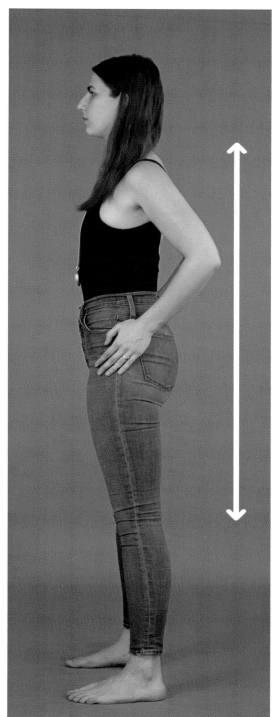

Exaggerated posterior tilt of the pelvis

Neutral spine

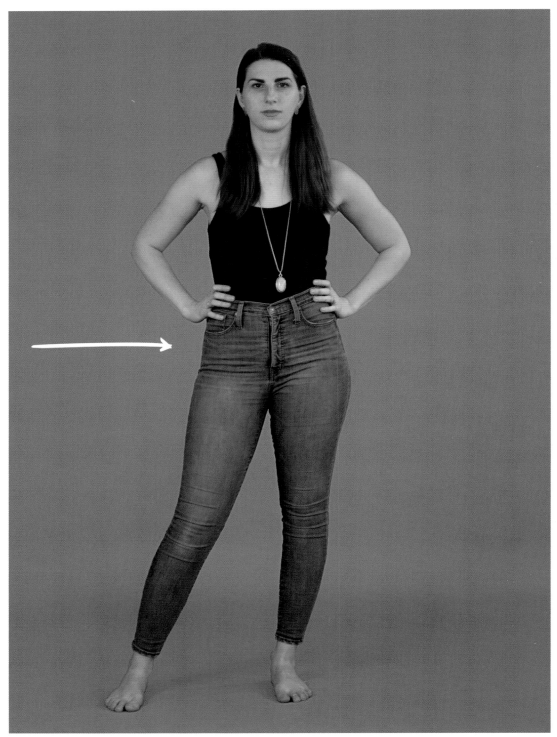

Leaning to one side creates a lateral tilt of the pelvis

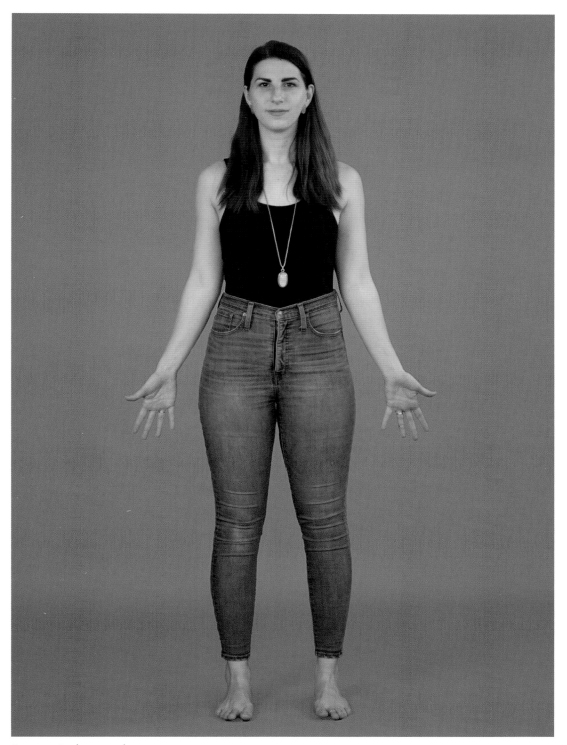

Anatomical neutral

Movement Break

Stand with your feet inner-hip-width apart. Make your feet parallel to one another like railroad tracks. Stand up tall and draw your shoulders back. Take note that when we adjust our posture, we often overcorrect. Pull your ribs in to bring your shoulders to a more neutral position. Tether your head back. Turn your palms forward and connect to your breath. Even when you are still, all the muscles in your body are working together to support you, resisting and assisting movement. Finding neutral can help you learn to counterbalance your most common movement patterns and learn new postures.

So how do you actually use anatomical neutral as a reference point in the studio if you have to look down at your work? The goal is not to stay in "perfect" alignment all day long. The main idea is to create good body mechanics as much as possible. Body mechanics is maintaining good posture throughout your movements in order to reduce stress on your muscles, joints, and connective tissues.

You might find yourself rounding over your workbench or drawing table in order to look down or get closer to your art. When you round forward in awkward positions, you create uneven pressure throughout your back. Raise your table so that you can work comfortably in an upright position. Rather than rounding over, try using your entire body to distribute the weight more evenly from the ground up.

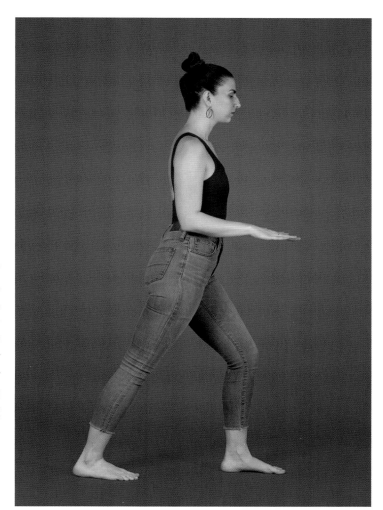

Lean in toward your workspace. Step one foot forward, as if to come into a lunge, and find a more neutral posture. Use your legs, lengthen your spine, and hinge at your hips to move toward your work rather than relying on your upper body to just hang there.

Movements of the Shoulder Blades

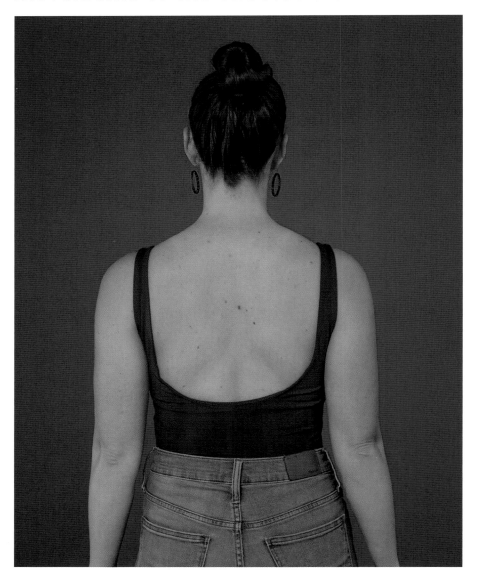

Neutral. The placement of your scapulae (shoulder blades) affects how you feel in your neck and shoulders. Understanding and practicing the different movements of the shoulder blades will help you find neutral throughout the day.

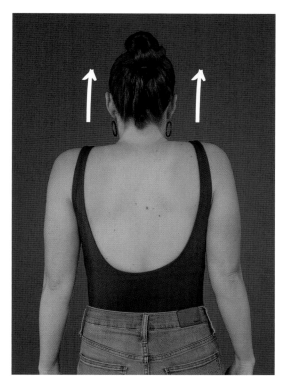

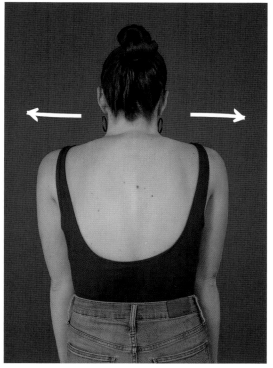

Elevation is the action of your shoulders moving up toward your ears. Do you tense up your shoulders when you're stressed out or worrying? I invite you to check in and relax your shoulders throughout the day.

Protraction (abduction) of the scapula is when your shoulders move away from your spine and round forward. Does this sound familiar? If you sit this way for long periods of time, the muscles in your back stay in an over-stretched position and need to build strength and stamina to learn new defaults.

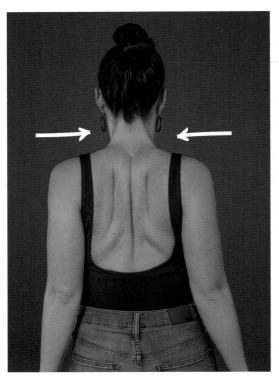
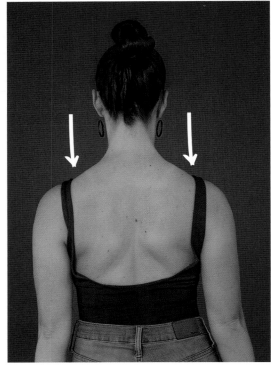

Retraction (adduction) is when your shoulder blades move back toward your spine. Retraction is the opposite of protraction. It's a great movement to practice in order to counterbalance the habit of rounding over your work. However, it is human nature to try to overcorrect! Which means you don't have to be in retraction all day long.

Depression is the action of your shoulder blades moving down your back. This movement can be helpful to practice if you are someone who sits or stands with their shoulders up toward their ears.

Movement Break

Now that you have more of an
understanding of the ways the shoulder
blades can move, take a moment to consider
which position you are in the most.
"Shoulder rolls" are a great exercise to target
your trapezius, rhomboids, and levator
scapulae muscles. Lift your shoulders up
toward your ears (elevation). Draw your
shoulder blades back toward your spine
(retraction). Lower your shoulder blades
down your back (depression). Pull your
shoulders forward to move your shoulder
blades away from your spine (protraction).
Engage with each position, work with your
breath, and roll with control. This exercise
has the ability to work out tension and
increase blood flow and circulation.

Seated Posture

This might come as a surprise, but it can be more physically challenging to keep an upright posture while sitting than standing. When you stand in a neutral position, the muscles of your hips work together with your trunk to keep you upright. As soon as you sit down, some of those muscles can no longer contribute as much, and your core has to compensate by working harder.

Sitting on an unpadded surface such as a folding chair will help you gain a more accurate understanding of the position of your pelvis. If your goal is to sit up tall and maintain a stronger neutral alignment for longer periods of time, checking in and readjusting is going to be critical no matter what type of chair you are in. As you learn what neutral alignment looks like while standing, you can use it as a reference to find neutral while sitting in whichever chair you have. It is important to be aware and consistently check in with your posture, readjust, and switch positions throughout the day.

Look at the following images. Which seated postures do you use while working in the studio? What does your posture look like when you readjust? Do you end up overcorrecting? We often don't realize what position we're in while we are working. It can be helpful to create a time-lapse video of yourself in the studio and come back to it to observe your movements. Compare the following images with your time-lapse video to have a clear idea of what your default positions and corrections look like. Making subtle adjustments will help retrain your muscles to create new patterns over time.

When you sit down, your legs have to bend far away from neutral, but your torso does not. Rounding in the upper back and jutting your head forward is just one way to get closer to your work. The other option is to sit with good body mechanics by keeping your torso closer to neutral and "hinging" forward from your hips.

Sitting well can be a challenge if you are not used to it, because when you slouch in the upper back, your tailbone has to round under to compensate. Developing more awareness of the position of your hips and bringing them closer to neutral can also make it easier to lengthen your spine and breathe more fully while you work.

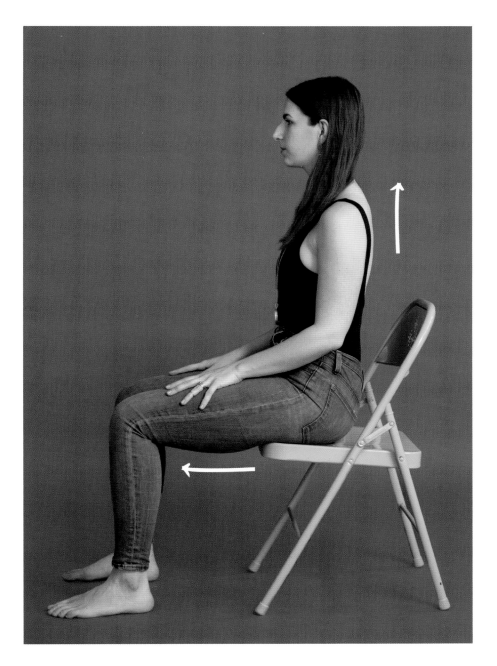

In a neutral seated position, your head, shoulders, and hips are vertically aligned. This allows your muscles, bones, and connective tissues to share the work of keeping you upright, so no one area gets overloaded.

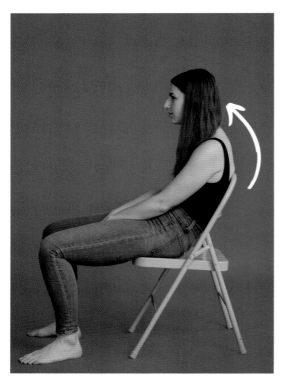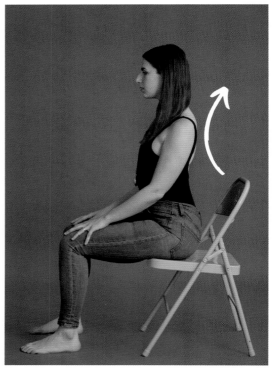

Exaggerated posterior tilt of the pelvis. Sitting too far forward in a chair in a relaxed position can force your pelvis to round under. This creates unnecessary tension on the low back.

An anterior tilt of the pelvis is when you lift your tailbone up and back. Overcorrecting in this way can force you into an exaggerated position, creating stress on the body.

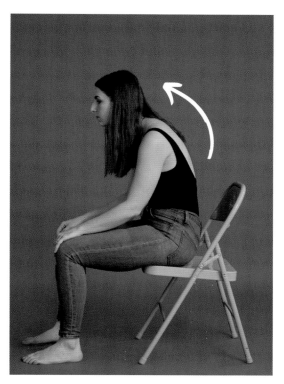

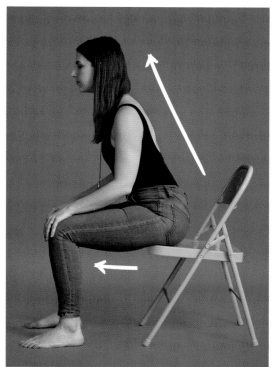

Shoulder protraction. When you round your shoulders forward, the shoulder blades will move away from your spine. This is called protraction. Excessive use of this position causes the back to overstretch and the pectoral muscles to tighten.

Position your artwork in front of you. "Hinge" at your hips.

Movement Break

Sit toward the front of your chair and align your knees directly over your ankles. Adjust the height of your chair so your thighs are parallel to the floor. Then sit up tall, keep your chin level, keep the back of your neck long, and readjust your shoulders. The action of readjusting your posture and activating your muscles will help you build strength in areas that are lacking. Press your feet down into the floor to distribute your weight more evenly. Create tension around your core muscles to stabilize the area. Activate the muscles in your back to help your shoulders find a more neutral posture. This practice can help you build strength and make it easier for you to sit well while you are working.

Sitting Affects Your Breath

Your breath is an incredibly amazing tool. We often take it for granted because it is always with us, but learning to breathe more mindfully can help you develop a deeper connection to your body and even help calm you down in times of stress.

Just like your heart beats day and night to keep your blood moving, your diaphragm and other breathing muscles are constantly working to pump air into and out of your lungs. You can build kinesthetic awareness of the movements of these muscles and learn to breathe in different ways. The common thread with abdominal breathing exercises is that they can activate your body's "rest and digest" response.[5]

When you are hunched over, there is less space in your chest cavity and abdomen for your lungs to expand, so your breathing will be shallow compared to the full capacity of your lungs. It is easier to breathe fully when you are standing or sitting with a more neutral alignment because it allows all the muscles woven through your torso to participate in expanding your lungs in all directions.

Cross-Legged Seated Posture

When you cross your legs while sitting in a chair, your pelvis will shift naturally to one side. This forces your body out of neutral. If you try to sit up tall, your spine will have to compensate by curving back the opposite way to bring your torso and head toward your midline.[6] The muscles on one side of your torso move into a shortened and compressed position, and the muscles on the other side become lengthened and can get overstretched. So it's no surprise that if you stay in this kind of position for hours at a time and then sit upright, you might feel tired, sore, or destabilized. These movements are not bad in small doses, but it's important to be aware of how they affect your body.

Remember that making small adjustments consistently can create a big difference. Every time you readjust, your muscle memory improves and you can notice something new about how you feel in your body, but it still takes time to develop new postural habits. If you love crossing your legs, it's okay! I am not telling you to toss out any one movement entirely. Instead, you can try crossing your feet at your ankles to keep your pelvis level. You can also use sitting with your legs crossed as an opportunity to add more variety to your day. Set an alarm to go off every fifteen minutes as a reminder to change your position. On the first alert: switch sides. On the second: come to neutral. On the third: get up and walk around.

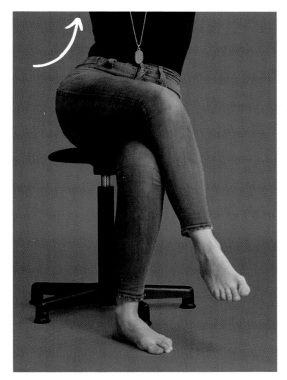
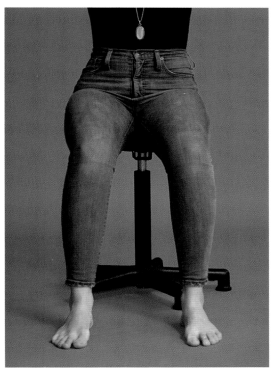

Sitting with your legs crossed tilts your pelvis to the side.

Neutral legs make it easier to sit up well.

Sitting with your legs crossed isn't the only way to move your pelvis out of neutral. Actions such as sitting on your phone or wallet can have negative effects on your structural health. Artists who use pedals to create their work are often affected by these movements. In this image, you will notice that my foot is raised onto a yoga block. This is an intentional exaggeration in height to give you an idea of the lateral movement that happens in the pelvis when an artist uses a foot pedal for extended periods of time. Potters often use a pedal to throw at the wheel, while jewelers or sculptors might use one to work with a flex shaft or Dremel tool. Even a small tilt to one side shifts your body out of a neutral alignment.

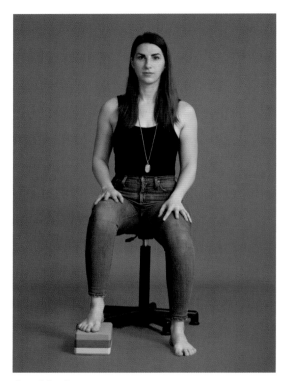

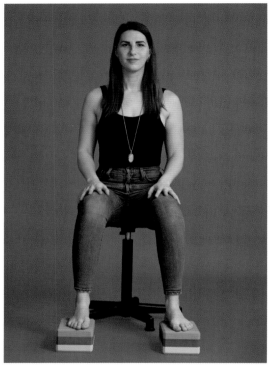

One block   Two blocks

Here, I am leveling the pelvis position by using a prop. A yoga block is great in this case; however, it might not be the correct height for what you need. The goal is to find something that is closest in height to the side that is elevated. Options may include a yoga block, a yoga wedge, books, a piece of wood, a brick, etc. Additionally, if neither of your feet touch the floor, adding props can bring the floor to you! This will keep your feet from dangling and allow you to evenly distribute your weight.

Movement Tracker

Take note of your movement breaks throughout the day. Remember that movement means to change position. Stand up, stretch, walk around, dance, wiggle, and switch tasks often. Trust me, your body will thank you!

MONDAY	TUESDAY
WEDNESDAY	**THURSDAY**
FRIDAY	**SATURDAY**
SUNDAY	**TAKEAWAYS**

Walking

Having good posture alone is not enough to keep you feeling great. It is extremely important to keep your muscles and joints moving. If you have good posture but don't move in different ways often enough, you can cause yourself a lot of discomfort. Walking is a gentle way to break up extended periods of sitting or standing.

Now that you've spent some time considering your standing and seated postures, I invite you to notice how your default positions influence the way you walk and move throughout the day. Note that the position of your feet and ankles affects the alignment in your joints from the ground up, which can compromise your ability to access a neutral position.

Even a small amount of internal or external rotation can create a lot of unnecessary pressure on your ankles, knees, hips, and so on.

Once you observe the alignment of your feet, take note of your ankles' tendencies. Do they cave in (pronation), or do you shift your weight to the outer edge of your foot and ankles (supination)? Our feet and ankles are meant to move in these directions, but when we hold these positions excessively, it can become problematic for the whole kinetic chain.

If it's hard for you to stand still for long periods of time this is your body's way of providing you with a signal. This is an opportunity to reevaluate your movement patterns in your feet and ankles. I struggled with pronation (ankles caving in) for many years. It was my default. This made it incredibly difficult and often painful for me while I was in graduate school for fine art. During critiques, we would stand for hours on hard flat surfaces. It was so challenging for me to stand for extended periods of time because my back would hurt pretty quickly. The pain would cause me to try to readjust but I couldn't hold an upright posture for long enough without getting uncomfortable. By the end of the day, I would be exhausted which impacted my productivity levels and mood. I really wish I knew then how much the alignment in my feet and my footwear impacted how I felt throughout my body.

Look at the following images and check in with your default. Notice the alignment of your feet, where the weight is distributed, and how your knee joint may be affected. You may be over-pronating if you are having trouble standing for long periods of time resulting in back and foot pain. Excessive pronation can lead to weakness in the gluteal muscles, also known as your butt! The

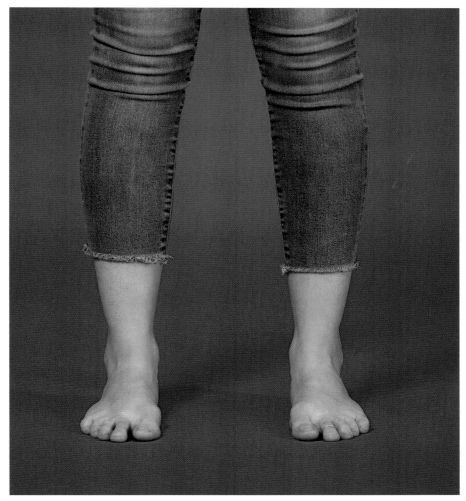

Neutral feet and ankles

gluteal muscles are incredibly important when it comes to keeping yourself upright in activities like walking, standing, and lifting. They help support our backs and so much more.

Another sign of pronation is if you look in a mirror and see that your knees knock inward while standing. Becoming aware of common misalignments will help you observe tendencies in your own movements. Start from the ground and work your way up! I invite you to reevaluate how you walk based on what you have observed about the way that you stand. Your walking habits were created slowly over the course of many years, so it is important to remember that creating new patterns takes time and consistent effort.

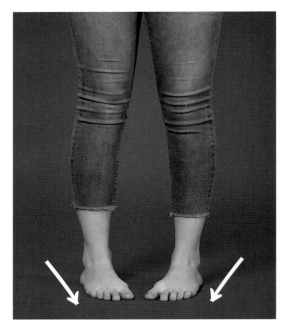

Feet turned in, also known as "pigeon-toed"

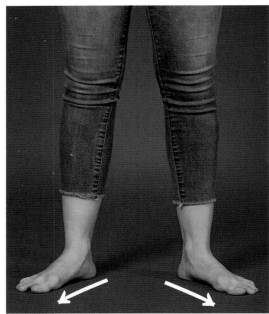

Feet turned out

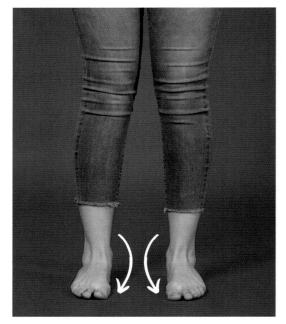

Pronation of the ankles forces the knees to cave in toward each other. This creates instability in the knees.

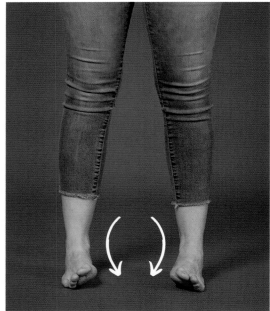

Supination of the ankles creates unnecessary strain on the joints.

Movement Break

Observe your feet and ankles. Do your feet turn in or out while you walk? Take a moment to notice what feels the most natural. We tend to think of our feet as parallel, but our defaults pull them out of neutral, especially while we are moving. For example, if you are used to walking with your feet externally rotated, turning your feet parallel can feel like an internal rotation. This is why it is critical to study your walking patterns. Take a lap around your studio space and then journal about what you observe. How much effort is it to walk with your feet parallel?

Footwear

What type of shoes do you wear while working in the studio? Most shoes have a heel, whether it's a comfortable pair of sneakers, work boots, or dress shoes. Standard shoes with even a small heel can shift your feet and ankles out of a neutral alignment. This forces the rest of your body to compensate for the misalignment by crafting new muscle patterns that can create instability and reduce ankle range of motion.

Do your shoes ever feel tight? Squeezing your toes into crunched positions is not the best option when it comes to structural health. Your feet are your foundation, and their alignment affects the rest of your body. They are too often overlooked or neglected. Your feet deserve a change of pace!

Minimal or "barefoot" shoes are designed to help you build strength in your feet and ankles rather than relying on a support to hold you up. The arch in regular shoes trains the muscles in your feet to relax, which makes it harder for them to go to work when you need them most. Minimal shoes are different from regular shoes in a few ways, and they can help you build more strength in your arch. They are zero drop, which means they have no heel. They have a much-wider toe box, which gives your whole foot room to stretch (you can even wear toe spacers with many of them). They also allow your feet to feel and respond to more variety in the terrain you walk on, which activates your muscles in a different way. The soles of your feet are covered with sensory receptors. Stimulating them with barefoot walking strengthens body awareness, improves balance and coordination, and promotes proper posture. Minimal shoes can be a great step on the path to developing more-resilient ankles![7]

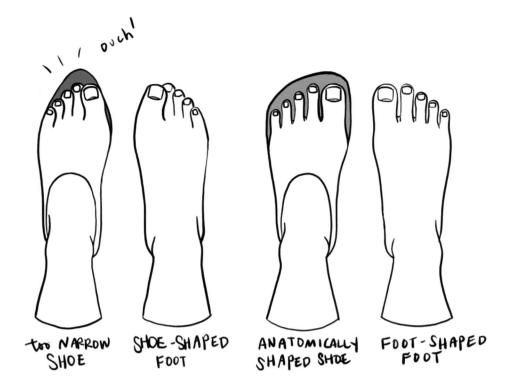

too NARROW SHOE

SHOE-SHAPED FOOT

ANATOMICALLY SHAPED SHOE

FOOT-SHAPED FOOT

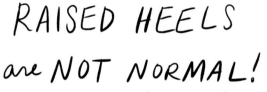

RAISED HEELS are NOT NORMAL!

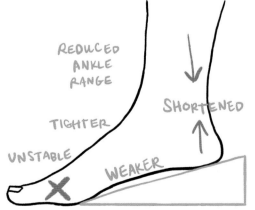

REDUCED ANKLE RANGE

SHORTENED

TIGHTER

UNSTABLE

WEAKER

Movement Break

Take a moment to pull out a few pairs of your favorite shoes. Look at the sole of each one. Are some areas worn down more than others? The inner edge, outer edge, heel, or toe? This will provide you with visual information about your walking patterns, which area of the foot you rely on the most, and if you depend on one foot more than the other.

Pain and Burnout

There is a fine line between hustle and burnout, and we live in a society that celebrates fatigue, stress, and tension as signs of hard work and success. So it's not surprising that we often ignore pain and overwork ourselves in order to "power through." Consider your own work habits. Have you ever sat in a chair for a long period of time, felt an uncomfortable sensation brewing in your body, and ignored it? Maybe it went away for a moment or two and then intensified. This is your body's way of signaling that you need to readjust, move around, or rest.

> "Do not overwork or ignore pain. I overworked. I love my life as a potter, but I overdid it, often working beyond fatigue and pain." —John Glick, *To Sciatica and Back: A Potter's Journey,* 1987

Pain is a broad term that refers to any uncomfortable sensations that you experience in your body. Studies show that individuals can respond to the same painful stimulus in different ways. For some, pain is distracting and negatively affects their performance on a task. For others, engaging with a task can be a way of staying distracted from pain, and the experience of pain can actually improve their performance up to a point. Finally, some respond to pain by sending their minds wandering.[8]

We often think of pain as a bad thing. However, it can be something positive if we recognize it as the body's way of communicating with us. If you choose not to listen to the signals that your body provides you with, they will get louder and louder until it's too much to ignore or an injury occurs.

> "Pain is always protective. Pain was preempted by a loss of stability or security somewhere, and each of us have a unique pain expression in the body." —Omni Kitts-Ferrara, *Pain and Movement,* 2020

I invite you to create a deeper dialogue with your body. Discomfort can be an early warning sign and an opportunity to engage differently or counterbalance the movements that are causing the issue. Recognize when it is time to readjust, to stand up, to move, or to rest. Take a movement break when it feels the most natural or needed. Journal about your experience, and notice if you begin to see an improvement with how you feel throughout the day.

Movement Tracker

Take note of your movement breaks throughout the day. Remember that movement means to change position. Stand up, stretch, walk around, dance, wiggle, and switch tasks often. Trust me, your body will thank you!

MONDAY	TUESDAY
WEDNESDAY	**THURSDAY**
FRIDAY	**SATURDAY**
SUNDAY	**TAKEAWAYS**

Movement Tracker

Take note of your movement breaks throughout the day. Remember that movement means to change position. Stand up, stretch, walk around, dance, wiggle, and switch tasks often. Trust me, your body will thank you!

MONDAY

TUESDAY

WEDNESDAY

THURSDAY

FRIDAY

SATURDAY

SUNDAY

TAKEAWAYS

STUDIO MOVEMENTS & MISALIGNMENTS

CHAPTER 4

When I first began my journey of finding neutral and maintaining good alignment, it was a huge challenge for me to sit up tall for thirty seconds. I would collapse after ten to fifteen seconds and fall back into my default position.

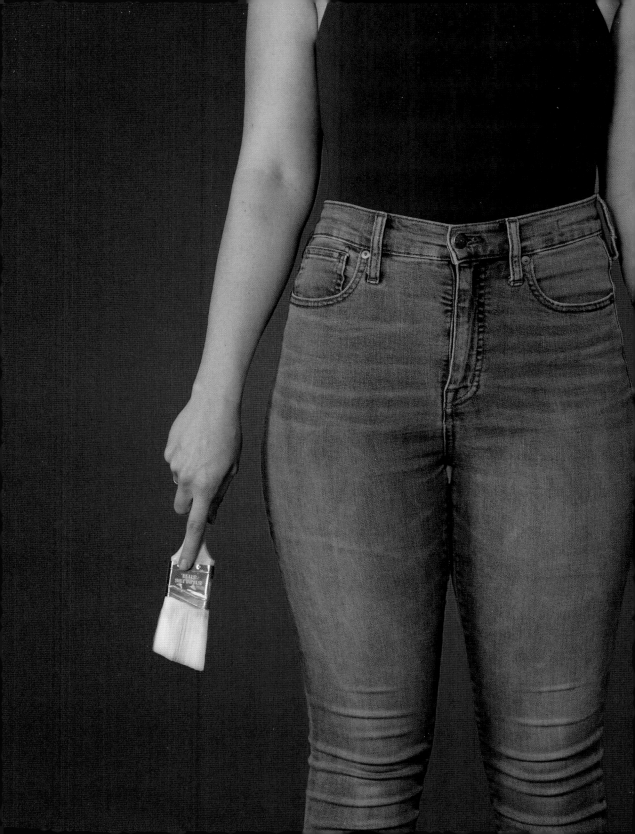

There were numerous events where I tried to sit well during a critique, workshop, or lecture and felt so uncomfortable. I remember feeling like I just couldn't do it. Like many, I adopted the phrase "I have terrible posture." It's not that I had terrible posture. It's that I wasn't crafting sustainable movement patterns. Like any other new skill, I had to take the time to learn new ideas and put in the effort to build kinesthetic awareness to advance the practice.

Consider a technique you use the most. Every time you repeat it, you are building muscle memory whether or not you have good form. At the end of the day, using the technique creates results in your artwork and in your body at the same time. If you are not happy with the outcome, you might practice the technique until you can create a result that reflects your creative vision. You are capable of learning new skills and movements. You have the same opportunity to reinforce positive or negative work habits by making small adjustments on a consistent basis.

Compensation Patterns

In order to create more-resilient movement patterns, it is important to recognize where you might be compensating. A pattern of compensation is created as the body's attempt to make up for a lack of mobility or strength in one area by relying on a different movement. These patterns arise for many reasons, including injuries, daily activities, or sitting in a chair for long periods of time. Compensation patterns can develop so slowly that we don't notice them until they've been around for quite a while. Unfortunately, if you are not mindful of the way you engage with repetitive movements, overuse and strain can cause new patterns of compensation that disrupt your other basic human movements and increase your risk of injury over time.[1]

When you think about creating a new movement pattern in your body and studio practice, remember that it requires patience and consistency. Your body has its own defaults and has been moving in particular ways for many years. It's important to recognize that you are not going to be able to change a pattern in just one try. It takes time, conscious effort, and patience with yourself to repeat the new movement enough for it to feel natural.

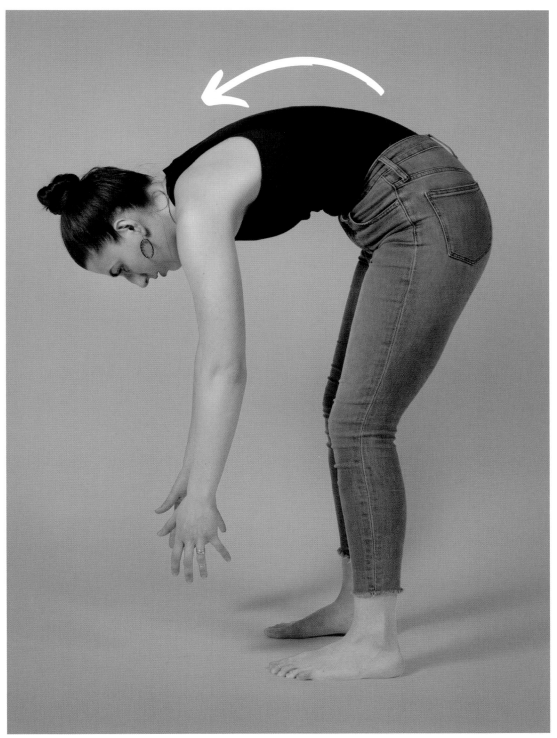

Forward fold with a rounded back

Folding

It is a common misconception that a muscle has to "relax" in order to stretch. When an external force is provided, like gravity in a forward fold, it is considered a passive stretch. If you go to do a forward fold and you round forward, chances are you will feel the stretch primarily in your back rather than your legs. This is because your back takes on the load in order to compensate for the lack of engagement in your legs and hips. If you push yourself into a stretch that your body is not ready for, you risk tugging on where the muscle meets the bone rather than stretching the belly of the muscle. This type of stretching can become counterproductive.

I encourage you to try a more active forward fold in order to gain more mobility. Rather than just rounding your back, bend your knees until you can touch the floor (or use props), push your feet down into the ground, hug your thighs in toward your midline, and create length in your spine. If you feel the stretch in your back, that is your body's way of signaling that your spine is taking on the load instead of your leg muscles.

I would rather you learn how to stretch in a way that builds strength and mobility than push yourself to get to the deepest version of a pose. When you push yourself too hard even in something like a forward bend, you risk continuing a compensation pattern in your body that is not sustainable. Just hanging there adds stress to your already overstretched back and puts you at risk of destabilization. But it doesn't have to be that way. Bend your knees. Feel the stretch in your legs. Lengthen your spine and breathe. Remember that the key to developing any new skill is consistency!

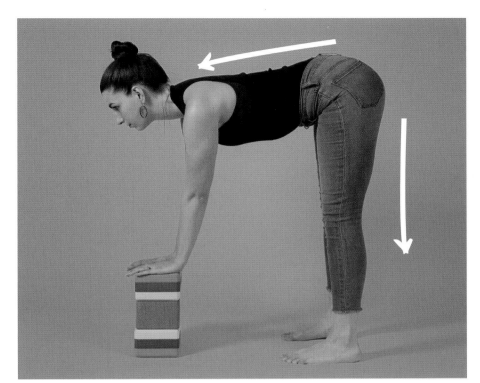

Forward
fold with
props,
straight legs,
and length-
ened spine

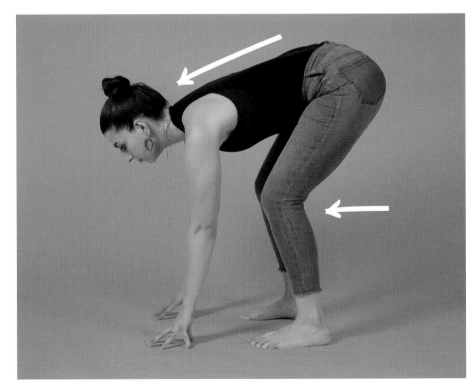

Forward
fold with
bent knees
and length-
ened spine

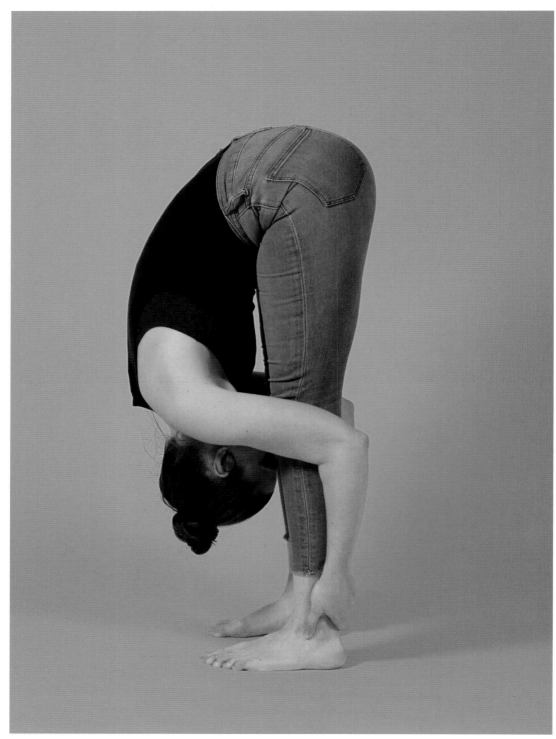

Advanced forward fold

Lifting

Have you ever experienced a pain signal while picking something up off the ground? Lifting concerns are often associated with picking up heavy objects, so we are usually more attentive and cautious compared to picking up everyday objects. Your body is a dynamic structure, and studies have shown that individuals with a healthy spine can safely pick up lighter items by either squatting or stooping to lift.[2]

When the weight of the object you need to lift (or its distance away from you) increases, the forces on specific areas of your spine can multiply. When you move carelessly, the weight will not distribute evenly through your body. Twisting while lifting can be especially dangerous, so it is important to be conscious of your movements.[3] Using good alignment to pick up smaller objects will help prepare your body so you can safely perform the movement pattern with a higher load.

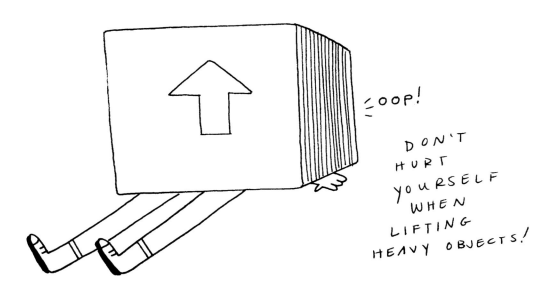

OOP!

DON'T HURT YOURSELF WHEN LIFTING HEAVY OBJECTS!

Introducing Squatting

How often do you squat down low to the ground? Squatting is a foundational movement that we naturally use while we're learning to walk. After being introduced to traditional chairs, we are encouraged to sit in them for long periods of time, and we are less inclined to squat throughout the day. Ultimately, it becomes more difficult to access. Since the movements and positions involved in squatting take you so far away from neutral, it is important to focus on strengthening within the range of motion that is safe for you. Start slow and listen to the signals your body provides you with.

When you sit in a chair, your hips are typically in 90 degrees of flexion for extended periods of time. The muscles that are responsible for flexing your hips are still active when you are sitting (all of your muscles are always working together to support you), but sitting does not require them to engage very much. In the same way, your gluteal muscles don't have to do much while you sit, and the connective tissues, nerves, and blood vessels in that area get compressed. This compression leads to decreased circulation and nerve signaling, which is why it is important to break up the posture and counterbalance a few times every hour.

If you are not exercising range of motion in your legs and hips regularly, it becomes more difficult to stand with a neutral pelvis. Incorporating squatting movements back into your everyday practice is a great way to exercise range of motion in your legs, hips, and ankles while bringing more awareness to the alignment of your pelvis. Accessing a squat is going to look a little different for everyone. In the following images, I show a few modifications for accessing a squat. Remember there is always more to try as you deepen your movement practice.

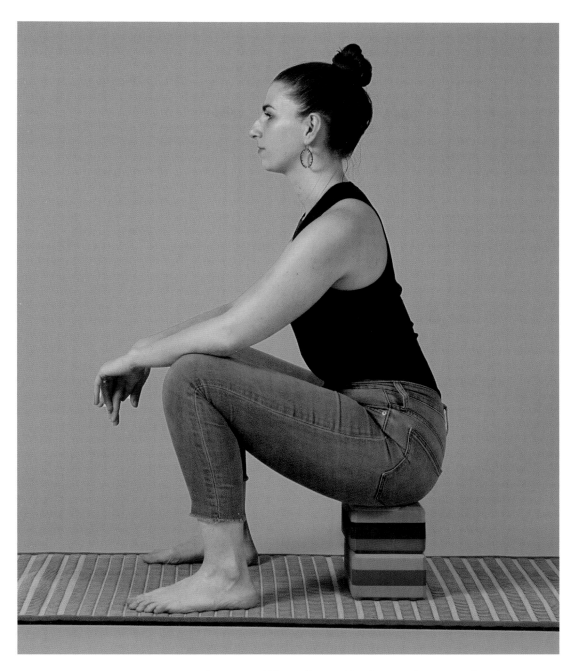

Supported Deep Squat: Get low to the ground and use props so you can lengthen your spine.

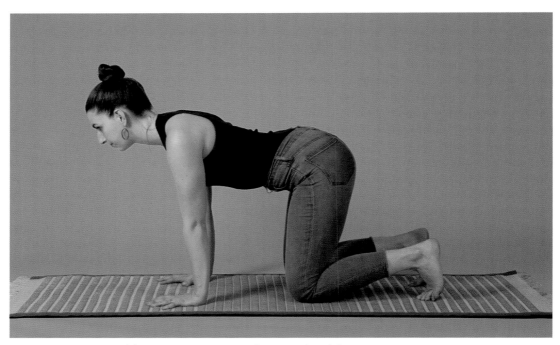

Step 1: Come to tabletop position. Stack your shoulders over your wrists. Position your hips over your knees. Tuck your toes under.

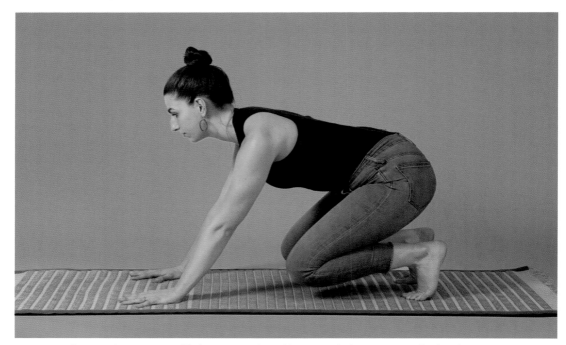

Step 2: Lift your knees up off the ground and hover. Shift your weight back toward your heels. Hold. Repeat steps 1 and 2 for a few rounds.

Movement Break

Lie on your back. Bend your knees, and place your feet on the floor underneath them. Notice the position of your tailbone by switching between a posterior and anterior tilt. In a posterior tilt, your tailbone will begin to peel up off the floor (imagine a scared dog who tucks its tail). In an anterior tilt, your tailbone will begin to point down toward the floor and create more space between your low back and the floor. Find a more neutral position between the two. There will still be a small amount of space between your low back and the floor.

From there, lift your feet and knees to 90 degrees. Check in with your pelvis. Begin to draw your knees toward your chest. The tendency is to begin to curl into a ball. Instead, use the floor as a prop to notice the position of your tailbone. Bring your knees in only until your tailbone would begin to lift (posterior tilt). Take a few breaths in this position. Over time, you can use this movement break to develop range of motion in your legs and more kinesthetic awareness of your hips and pelvis.

Making

Did you know that the muscles of your forearms are in charge of moving and stabilizing your wrists and fingers? Learning more about the way you move will be beneficial for your overall health and well-being. Your wrists can move in a variety of ways. Some examples include extension, flexion, abduction, adduction, and neutral positions. Look at the following images and consider which movements look the most familiar for your process.

A potter who throws at the wheel all day or wedges clay for long hours might find their wrists in extension, whereas a weaver might notice their wrists moving in adduction while working at the loom. It is important to build the habit of keeping neutrality in your wrists, especially when you are working in the studio. Overuse, force, and time away from neutral can lead to inflammation in the area and compression on your median nerve, which can lead to carpal tunnel syndrome. This kind of compression can also happen if you often rest your wrists or forearms on a hard surface, such as the edge of a table or workbench. Finding and maintaining a more neutral wrist position and learning how to use your hands, wrists, and forearms more effectively can be liberating.[4]

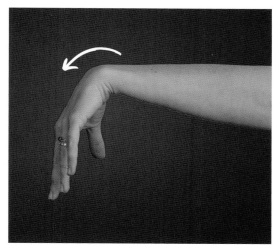

Flexion

Extension

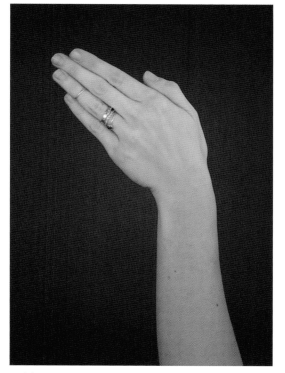

Adduction

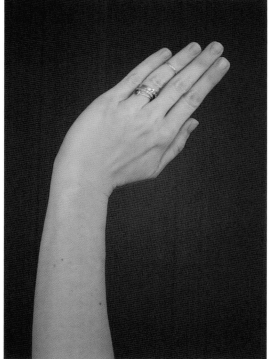

Abduction

Movement Break

What position are your wrists in the most throughout the day? Slowly move your wrists through flexion and extension. Take a moment to counterbalance the action you find yourself in the most with a stretch. Extend your right arm out in front of you, with your palm facing down. Use your left hand to gently bend your right wrist in toward you (flexion) until you feel a stretch in your forearm. Hold there for three deep breaths. Release your right hand and turn your palm up. Use your left hand to gently bend your right wrist down and back toward you (extension) until you feel a light stretch. Hold for three deep breaths and then switch sides.

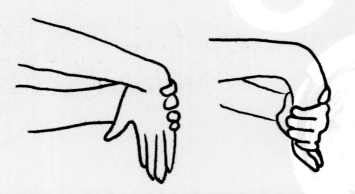

Pinching

Pinching and gripping is a lot of work for the muscles and joints of the hands, wrists, and forearms. Do you depend on your pointer finger or thumb to create precise pressure, or do you evenly distribute the pressure by using your entire hand? One position isn't necessarily better than another; it is just important to recognize where you can create more variety in your movements. Remember that choosing the same action over and over again makes it more likely that you will develop a repetitive strain injury. So pick up a tool, hold it in a few different ways, and try something a little new. Creating variety in your movements can open up possibilities and will benefit your practice over time.

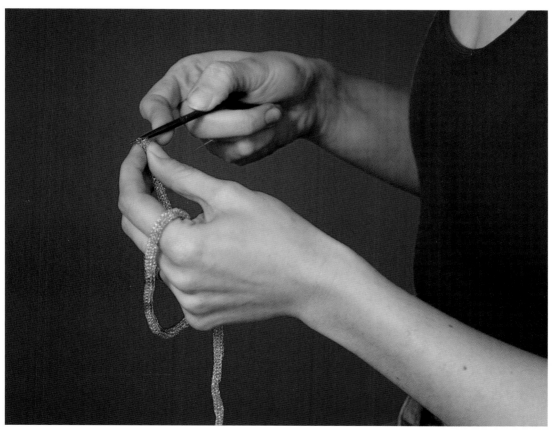

In this image, I am knitting silver wire. My pointer finger's first knuckle holding the tool (right hand) is in hyperextension.

When you use your pointer finger to pinch or press, does your first knuckle go into hyperextension? Hyperextension in your fingers can happen when you lock a knuckle joint to apply pressure. If the force pushes your finger sideways instead, it is called lateral deviation. Techniques that involve these movements need to be performed carefully and with enough support for the vulnerable joints. When a joint gets pushed beyond its range of motion in any direction, the ligaments around it can be overstretched or damaged and the nerves in the area can become compressed. Use your fingers more mindfully by adding a micro bend to bring the joint closer to neutral. This may be more challenging at first, because the muscles of your hands, wrists, and forearms have to manage the load that was on the ligament, and it will take time to retrain your muscle memory.

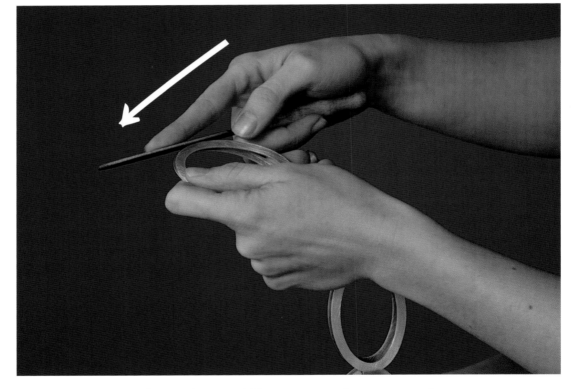

In this image, I am working with a metal file. My pointer finger is not in hyper-extension, and I am maintaining a more neutral position. As you work with your tools (files, pencils, paintbrushes, needles, etc.), use the strength of your hands, wrists, and forearms to maintain more neutrality while pinching and gripping.

Strengthening exercises increase muscle tone, which is important for creating health in your carpal tunnel region. The best way to strengthen your hands, wrists, and forearms is to counterbalance the motions you do the most. If you are constantly gripping tools, think about how you can introduce a new movement to create more balance over time.

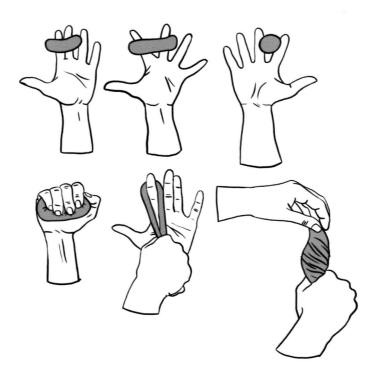

Therapy putty is great for this type of action. It helps restore biomechanical balance to your hands, wrists, and forearms. Using therapy putty regularly will strengthen the muscles of your hands and arms in a different way. This can help relieve the strains that develop from overworking these muscles with repetitive motions.

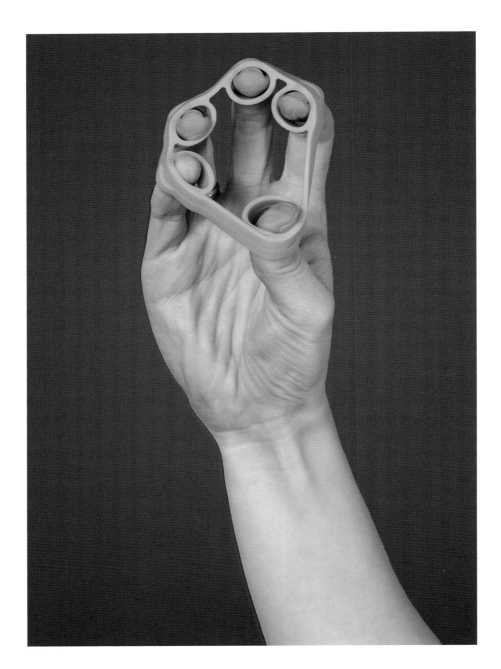

Strengthening tools are great for counterbalancing the actions of pinching and gripping. Place your fingers in the holes and position the band at the base of your fingertips. Slowly expand and contract for a few reps. Take your time and move slowly. A little bit goes a long way.

Movement Tracker

Take note of your movement breaks throughout the day. Remember that movement means to change position. Stand up, stretch, walk around, dance, wiggle, and switch tasks often. Trust me, your body will thank you!

MONDAY	TUESDAY
WEDNESDAY	**THURSDAY**
FRIDAY	**SATURDAY**
SUNDAY	**TAKEAWAYS**

CHAPTER 5 MENDING

A stitch in time may save nine.
—Anonymous, ca. 1733[1]

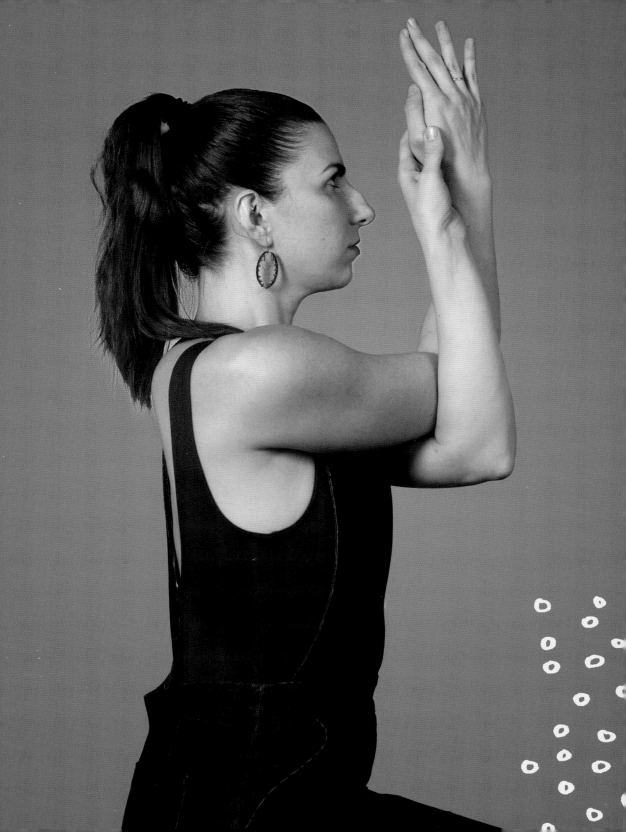

Have you ever sewed up an old pair of jeans? If you tear your pants or favorite shirt but still want to continue wearing it for a while, you will want to mend it before it gets worse over time. Repairing the issue early allows you to strengthen your garment so that it will last longer. Just like your belongings occasionally need tending to, your body needs to be strengthened in some areas and massaged in others in order to create longevity. Putting things off can cause you more harm than good. If you take the time to care for your body now through movement and massage, you are much more likely to improve the longevity of your practice. Learning how to incorporate massage, stretching, and strengthening techniques into your everyday practice in order to care for your body will inspire you to mend consistently.

What Is a Fascia?

If you've taken a fitness class, received a professional massage, or worked with a wellness professional, you might have heard the words "connective tissue" or "fascia" tossed around. I first learned about fascias during massage therapy school as a type of connective tissue that surrounds our muscles and binds our internal structures together. Many massage techniques are designed to help rehydrate the tissues in these areas so you feel less stiff. This is why it is important to drink additional water for massage techniques to have longer results. More-recent research has shown that all of the fascias in your body are actually one whole system.[2]

Fascias are woven through and surrounding your muscles, organs, and bones. Fascias contain touch receptors, so you have an internal system that is sensitive to pressure and movement just like your skin![3] Fascias provide structure and are designed to stretch and expand as you move. If you lack movement and circulation to an area, the fascia will have less fluid moving through it, and over time it can become less pliable. When you sit, the tissues in your legs become compressed and dehydrated. Cellulite is physical evidence of what sitting for long periods of time can do to your body and connective tissues.[4]

When an area of your body is compressed, the collagen fibers in the connective tissue can get knotted together, creating knots. While going to a spa to see a professional massage therapist is ideal, it's not always an option. The good news is you have the ability to mend and repair your body in order to keep your tissues healthy through movement and massage. Remember to move your body, stretch, and incorporate massage regularly.

Movement Break

If you sit for a lot of the day, try to reorganize your work space in a way that encourages you to get up and move around more often. For example, if you alternate between two tasks hourly that are at separate sides of the room, it forces you to get up, walk around, and get your blood flow moving! Consistently taking a one-to-two-minute movement break every half hour to get up and walk around can help restore your tissues. This can also be a great opportunity to drink some water so your body can stay hydrated throughout the day.

Sense of Touch

Did you know that touch is the first sense that we develop in the womb? Isn't that incredible? In order to experience touch, we have a huge network of nerve endings and touch receptors in the skin. These receptors send signals to our brain so we can understand the world and objects around us.

Consider the way you learn or the way you handle materials when you're creating. What is your process like in terms of touch? For me, as an artist, touch is an incredibly important aspect of my process because my artwork is primarily about my tactile understanding of the body. Exploring textures and materials helps me consider what I want the viewer to explore as they interact with my work. How important is the sense of touch in your process of making?

The system for your sense of touch is made up of multiple types of receptors:

Mechanoreceptors allow us to experience textures, pressures, and vibrations. You can stimulate these receptors by handling a material or object in your workspace. Or just notice the fabric of your clothing on your skin. Maybe notice your phone vibrate when you get a confetti text.

Thermoreceptors. These receptors perceive sensations related to the temperature of objects when they come in contact with the skin. So, understanding hot and cold. This receptor will be stimulated if you go to grab a hot or cold beverage, or maybe you're a jeweler and you go to pick up a hot piece of metal by mistake. Ouch!

Pain receptors. These detect pain that can cause physical damage to the skin or other tissues of the body. Self-explanatory, but think about a time your pain receptors went off today. It could be something like stubbing your toe or cutting your hand with a chisel in the studio.

And finally there are **proprioceptors,** which are found in the tendons, muscles, and joints. Their location allows you to detect changes in muscles length, muscle tension, and joint position. These are going to be stimulated when you go to stretch or move out of a position you've been in for a while.

Your touch receptors are not just skin deep! They are woven all the way through your muscles and connective tissues. When you are sitting or standing still, these receptors respond to tension around joints, as well as length or compression in muscles. When you are moving, they sense changes to compression and length to create awareness of how your body is moving itself.

Movement Break

I invite you to place your right hand on your heart and your left hand on top of your right. Close your eyes and connect to your breath. Notice the warmth of your hands. Maybe even the pressure and weight of your hands resting on your chest. Notice where any pain or discomfort might exist in your body, or if you need to move and make an adjustment. How do you feel? I invite you to pay attention to your sense of touch and notice what it's stimulated by.

Incorporating Massage

If you weren't trained as a massage therapist, chances are that your instinct is to use your thumb to massage your opposite hand. Implementing self-care in this way is actually counterproductive. One of the first things a professional massage therapist learns during training is to avoid using their already over-worked thumbs to apply pressure. So as a maker interested in incorporating this modality into your daily routine, I recommend rolling a soft foam ball between your hands instead. Remember that a little bit goes a long way! Your hands and your feet have a very thin layer of connective tissue, which means they don't require much pressure in order to find relief.

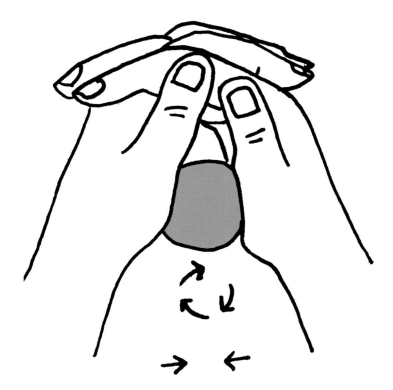

It's important to remember whenever you are practicing self-massage tech-niques to listen to the signals your body offers you. For example, if you are massaging a specific area and your muscles begin to clench or you are holding your breath, that is information that you are applying too much pressure. Ease off, connect to your breath, and apply less pressure.

If you work with your breath, you will get more out of the modality. Applying too much pressure can actually damage your connective tissue. If you notice that your breath and the intensity of the massage is increasing, that means that the pressure is too deep. If you are working with your breath and you notice that the intensity is decreasing, that means the area is releasing and the pressure is just right! That's why it is critical to gain a deeper connection to your body.

Massage Tools

Soft foam balls are a great way to incorporate massage into your daily practice. The layers of connective tissues in your hands are thin, which means they are ultimately more vulnerable to injury. You don't have to press hard in order to experience results. Light to medium pressure is enough to find relief.

Tennis balls are really inexpensive, accessible, and easy to find and carry around with you. They're a great way to begin incorporating self-massage. The density of the ball is not too hard, so they are often suggested by physical therapists to use for self massage. If you want a ball that will last longer that is specifically designed to support your body, I suggest the **Yoga Tune Up Fitness® Balls**. The balls come in a set of two with a pouch to carry them in. They are perfect for pinpointing specific areas.

Mini foam rolling is similar to traditional foam rolling, just mini! Foam rolling is widely practiced in athletic, rehabilitative, and home settings to improve range of motion, decrease soreness, increase blood flow and circulation, and relieve muscle pain. Large foam rollers are used to massage out larger areas of the body. Mini foam rollers can be used on the hands, wrists, and forearms to help hydrate your connective tissues and lubricate your joints. There are different types of mini foam rollers out there, but I find the RistRoller® to be most effective. You can even use it on your feet! This is a great tool to use throughout the day in your workspace.

Large foam rollers come in different sizes and densities. When used properly they can be a really great way to access temporary relief. Just like the density of balls mentioned above, if a foam roller is too firm it can actually do more harm than good. Massage tools are always going to feel more intense if you have to lay your body weight onto them, so it's important to remember that you don't need the firmest tool out there. I suggest finding a softer and more flexible option. If you can't bend it or compress it, it's probably too hard. A foam roller can be a great tool to use after a long day of working in the studio.

Massage is an incredible modality. Even short sessions of massage to move the muscle tissues, fibers, and fascias by hand or with a tool can encourage your body to release, reset, and even mend. I've curated a selection of tools on the Wellness for Makers website that I use in my practice and find the most beneficial. Use the following images to guide yourself through a series of massage techniques to find the relief you deserve.

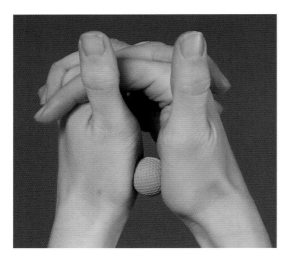 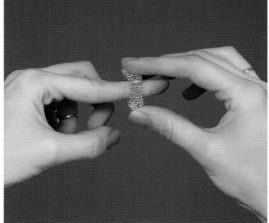

Soft foam massage balls feel great on your aching hands. Roll and compress the foam ball between your hands for a minute at a time. Pause on any areas that need a little extra love. This will help hydrate your connective tissues and lubricate the joints in your hands.

Acupressure rings help stimulate the acupressure points in your hands. They're also great for fidgeting! Place the acupressure ring on your finger and roll it up and down to increase blood flow and circulation. This is a gentle tool that is great for relieving stiff joints.

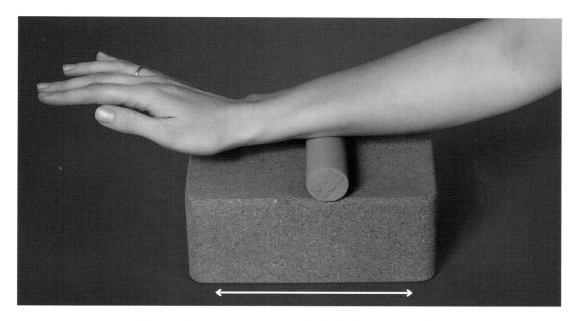

Mini foam rolling is a great way to find relief in your hands, wrists, and forearms. Place your roller on a hard surface (tabletop, block, or wall) and glide back and forth. Be sure to massage all sides of your hands, wrists, and forearms.

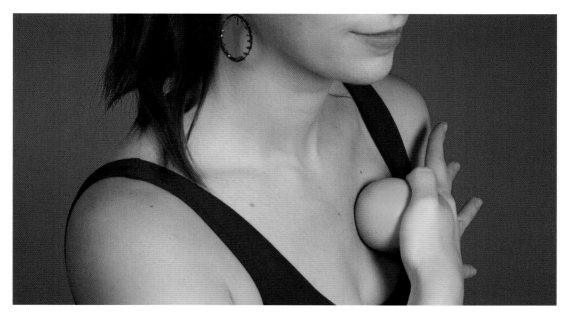

Massage balls are a great tool to use to massage out your pectoral muscles. Place the ball on the underside of your clavicle bone (also known as the collarbone). Gently glide the ball back and forth to relieve any tense areas.

Benefits of Massage

☐ Elongate muscles

☐ Increase blood flow and circulation

☐ Hydrate connective tissues

☐ Lubricate joints

Stretch

Typically when people think of stretching, they associate it with passive stretching. There are a variety of different types of stretching, but in this section, we will focus on passive vs. active stretching techniques.[5] You can get so much more out of the practice if you learn how to distinguish between them.

Passive stretching is when an external pressure is applied so a specific muscle can "relax" and be stretched at the same time. The force could be added from a strap, wall, partner, or even your own body weight. While passive stretches are fine in small amounts, they should be done with care or you can cause more harm than good. If you push yourself into a stretch that your body is not ready for, you can actually tug on where the muscle meets the bone rather than stretching the belly of the muscle evenly. This risks creating destabilization in the body.

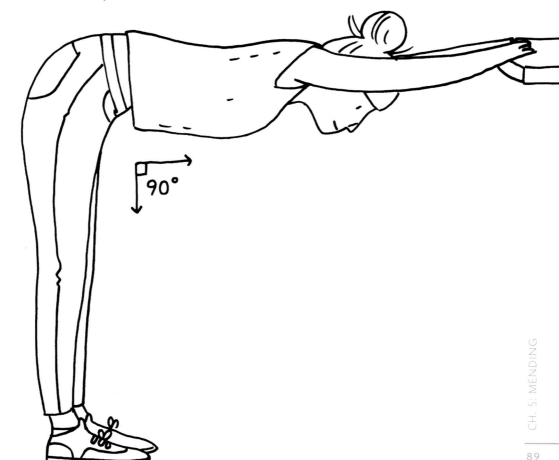

90°

Active stretching is when you co-engage your muscles to move or hold a position, including the muscles that are getting the stretch. This creates less of a chance for overstretching and helps you develop more mobility and stability. Active stretching is an effective way to build muscle strength and can lead to increased flexibility.[6]

The following exercises involve these concepts and can be performed while sitting or standing. This section is a great one to come back to throughout your workday. These movements are especially helpful to incorporate if you've been rounding over. As always, I encourage you to move slowly and listen to the signals your body provides you with. The goal of this section is to help you gain a deeper understanding of how to move your body through observation and action. Notice if you have a tendency to hold your breath during movement. Listen to your body's needs, honor its strengths and limitations, and readjust as needed.

Reach your right arm up toward the ceiling. Bend at your elbow and lower your hand behind you. Place your left hand on your right elbow. Press your elbow and hand into each other to create resistance. Connect to your breath.

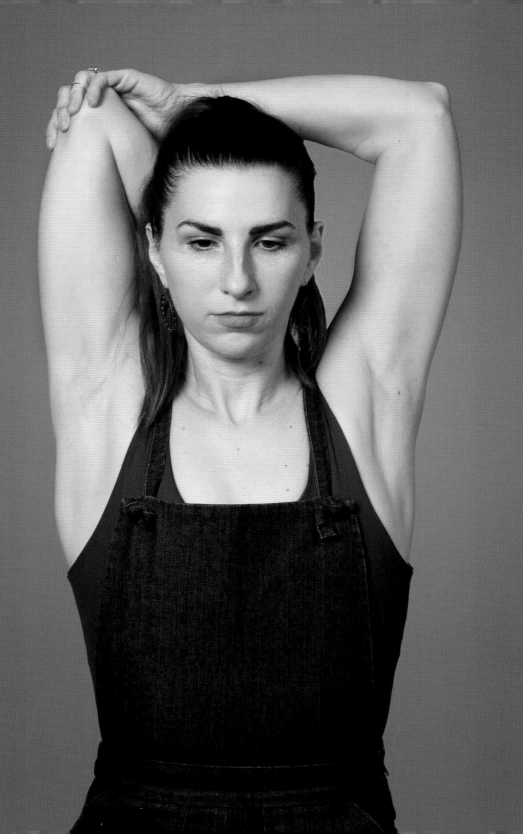

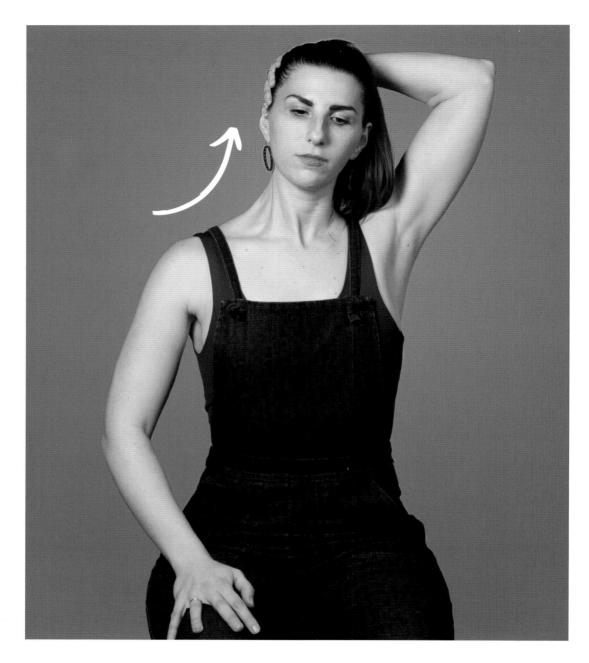

Lateral neck stretch: Place your right hand toward the back of the left side of your head. Tilt your head toward the right. The pressure from your hand will create a passive stretch. Rather than hanging there, activate the posture by pressing your head up and back into your hand.

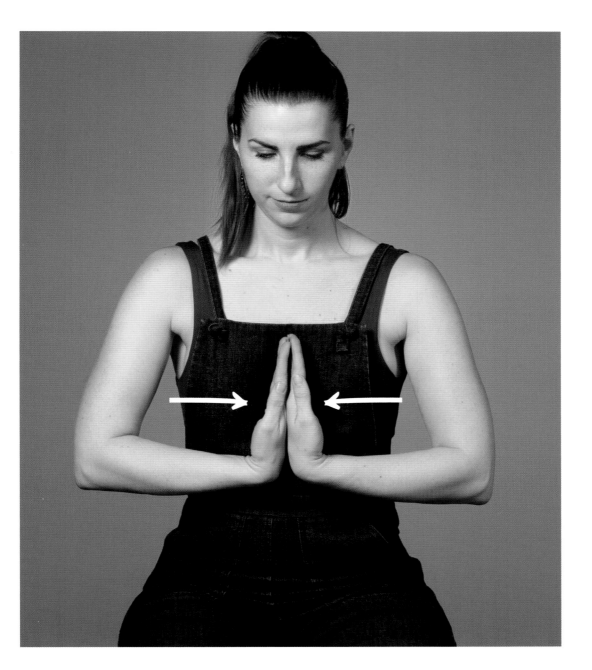

Reverse prayer wrist stretch: Bring the backs of your hands to touch until you feel a light stretch. Move your hands down to increase the pressure and up to decrease the pressure as needed. Please note that you may not have the same amount of flexibility as I do in this image and that's okay!

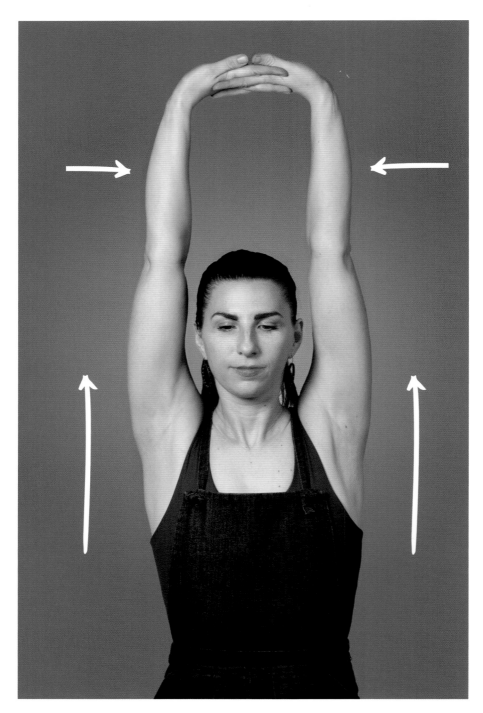

Latissimus dorsi stretch: Interlace your hands in front of you. Lift your arms up toward the sky. Hug your arms in toward each other and reach!

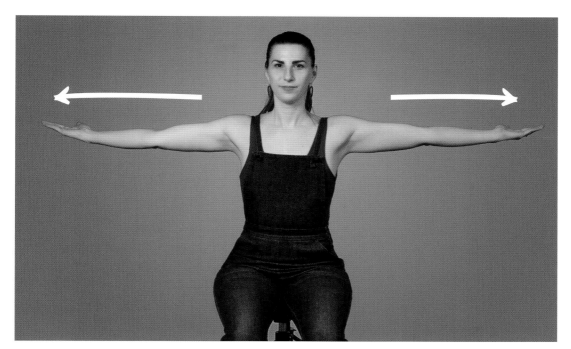

Stretch step 1: Extend your arms out to your sides. Turn your palms up toward the sky.

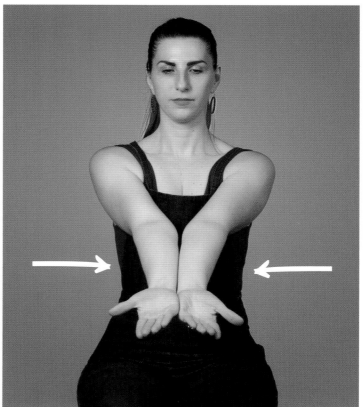

Stretch step 2: Bring your hands and pinkie fingers to touch and hug your forearms toward each other.

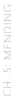

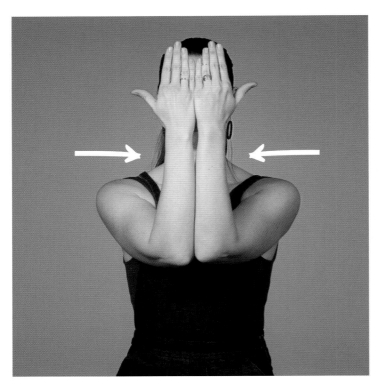

Step 3: Bend your elbows and lift your hands in front of your face. Hug your arms in toward each other to fire up your muscles. Lift your elbows up a little bit higher to increase the stretch, and lower your elbows to decrease the intensity.

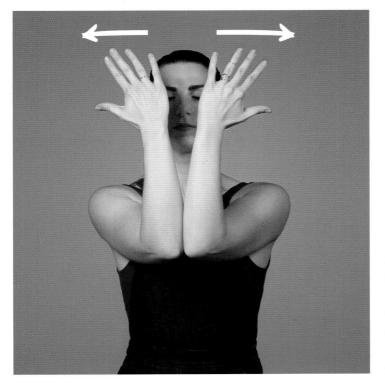

Step 4: Peel your fingers and hands apart. Take three deep breaths. Where do you feel the stretch? Near your shoulder blades, arms, pectoral muscles? Take note. Connect to your breath and release.

Benefits of Stretching

☐ Increase range of motion

☐ Reduce risk of injury

☐ Improve mobility

☐ Reduce pain and strain

Strength

Learning how, when, and where to actively engage your muscles will empower you in any movement. In the following exercises, I invite you to grab some props. I am using a light-to-medium-weight resistance band and a yoga block. If you don't have a yoga block, grab a book around the same size. Props are really helpful tools to guide you to build awareness in the body. These exercises can be performed sitting or standing. I am seated in the photos to remind you that you have the opportunity to bring more movement into your work space throughout the day. I do invite you to get up and move around as much as possible, and including the following movements is a great way to do so.

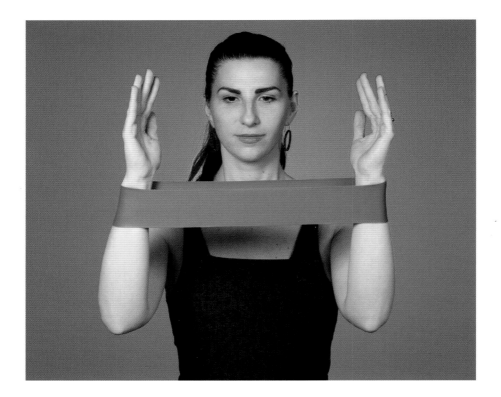

Resistance bands are a great way to strengthen your arms throughout the day. Thread your hands inside the band below your wrists. Sit up tall, slowly press your arms into the resistance band, and then release. Continue for a few reps.

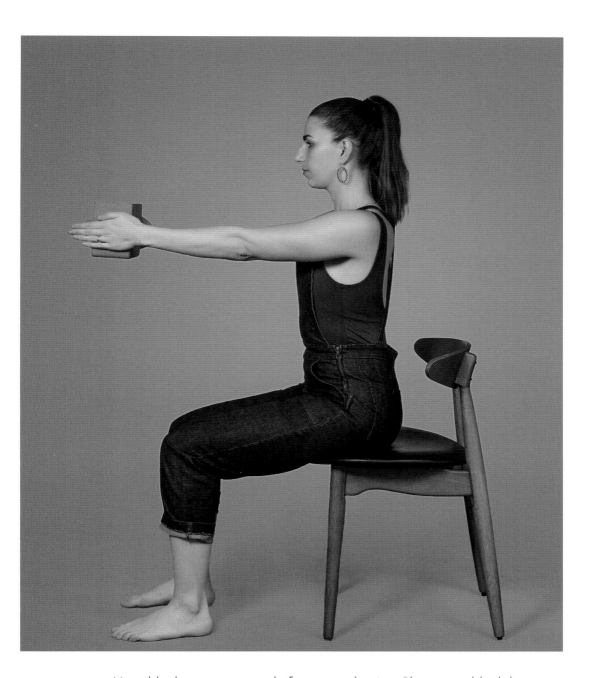

Yoga blocks are great tools for strengthening. Place your block between your hands and hold it out in front of you. Hug your hands in toward each other to create engagement in your arms.

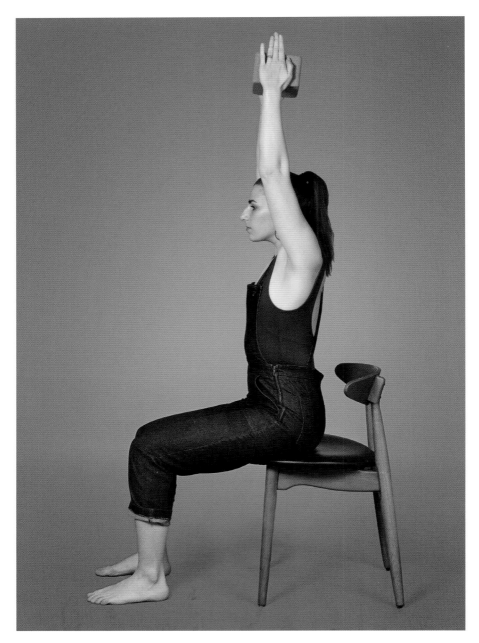

Squeeze your arms toward the block and slowly lift it up toward the sky. Notice if your elbows want to bend. Go only as far as you can while maintaining straight arms. Your mobility might look very different than mine does in this picture, and that's okay!

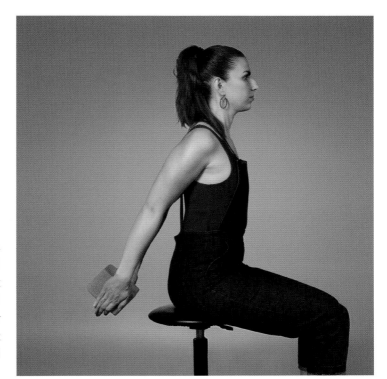

Extension of shoulders. This movement can be done seated or standing. Position the block between your hands behind you. Sit up tall. Open up your chest. Extend your arms back and hug your arms toward the block.

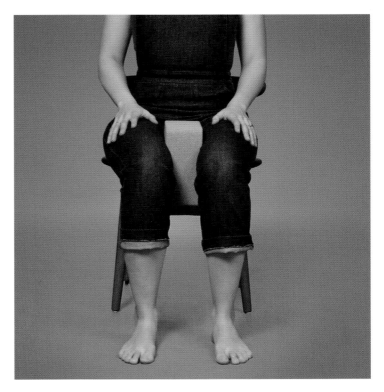

Blocks are great for bringing awareness to your inner thighs as well. Sit up tall and position your knees over your ankles. Place the block between your thighs and squeeze.

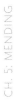

Benefits of Strengthening

☐ Increase muscle tone

☐ Improve alignment

☐ Create longevity

☐ Improve balance

Movement Tracker

Take note of your movement breaks throughout the day. Remember that movement means to change position. Stand up, stretch, walk around, dance, wiggle, and switch tasks often. Trust me, your body will thank you!

MONDAY

TUESDAY

WEDNESDAY

THURSDAY

FRIDAY

SATURDAY

SUNDAY

TAKEAWAYS

CHAPTER 6 STUDIO IMPROVEMENT

The way you move and how much movement you get throughout the day is heavily influenced by your studio setup. This includes how you arrange furniture, organize tools and equipment, select a chair, and more. Back in 2016, I interviewed studio potter Kristen Kieffer for the *Wellness for Makers* blog about her studio setup and standing at the wheel to throw.

Throughout our conversation, Kristen described her process as being "purposefully inefficient." She went on to explain that she intentionally changes positions, techniques, and tasks in order to reduce her risk of developing a repetitive strain injury in the future.

Take a moment to consider which parts of your practice are the most repetitive. Whether you are a potter, jeweler, woodworker, fiber artist, painter, etc., you might think that breaking up tasks will waste time in creating your piece, finishing an order, or preparing for your latest exhibition, but consider how much time could be lost if you were to end up out of work with an injury. If making is your passion, your livelihood, and your career, can you really afford to take such a risk?

"You don't have to sit down to knit. Knitting was created to be done on the go. It's an attempt to get us away from being seated at a loom."

—Carson Demers,
author of *Knitting Comfortably: Ergonomics of Handknitting*

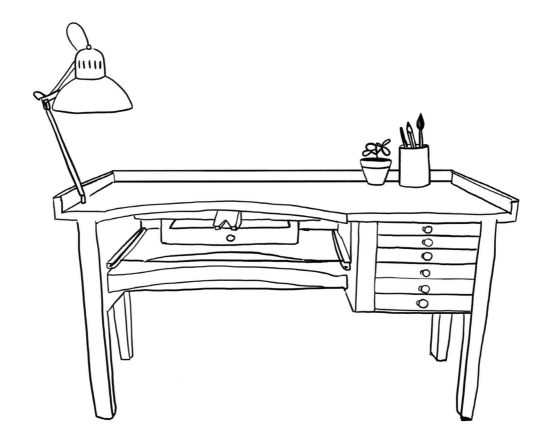

Are you prioritizing convenience over variety?

I encourage you to look at your studio setup and consider where you can create opportunities to vary your movements throughout the day. Try reorganizing tools and materials you use often, so you will reach up high, squat down low, or walk across the room, rather than keeping everything in the most convenient place. Create multiple workstations that encourage you to move differently. A space for sitting, standing, or even squatting. Which tasks can you do standing up, even for a few minutes at a time? Can you switch to an adjustable-height workbench, pottery wheel, or drawing table? Prioritizing convenience often leads to less variety in our movements throughout the day. Standing while working in the studio has the ability to shift your perspective and may even inspire a new body of work, depending on your process and what equipment you have available.

Which Chair Should I Use?

Have you ever wondered which chair is the best chair for your studio practice? Or whether or not to use a lumbar support or an ergonomic cushion? Artists ask me these things all the time. The answer is going to depend on you, your practice, and what you want to achieve in your body. While I do see the benefits of occasionally using lumbar support while working to retrain your muscles, it is important to remember that sitting well does not require a fancy ergonomic chair. You also don't have to sit in the same chair all day long or use the same ergonomic cushion for hours on end. Switch it up. Have options.

In my workshops, I typically use a traditional folding chair. If your goal is to sit up tall and maintain a stronger neutral alignment for longer periods of time, checking in and readjusting is going to be critical no matter what type of chair you are in. If you understand what neutral alignment looks like while standing, you can use that as a reference guide to find neutral while sitting in whichever chair you have. When you sit, the curvature of your spine affects the load force on the rest of your body. So it is important to be aware and consistently check in with your posture, readjust, and switch positions throughout the day.

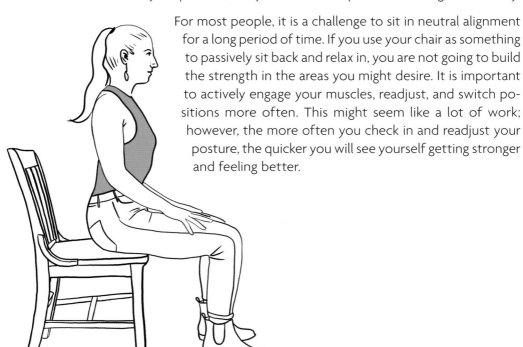

For most people, it is a challenge to sit in neutral alignment for a long period of time. If you use your chair as something to passively sit back and relax in, you are not going to build the strength in the areas you might desire. It is important to actively engage your muscles, readjust, and switch positions more often. This might seem like a lot of work; however, the more often you check in and readjust your posture, the quicker you will see yourself getting stronger and feeling better.

Chair Alternatives

One of the major themes of this book is that it's important to move around as much as possible. So having a few options in the studio is the key to creating more-diverse movement patterns. I find that switching positions often is very beneficial. Rather than depending on one posture all of the time, switch it up! Try moving from a chair, to standing, to a stability ball, to kneeling, to a squatting position. I have a few props that I use to help me increase the amount of movement I engage with throughout the day.

The Soul Seat is a nontraditional chair that invites you to move around from shape to shape. The "perch" is inspired by a yoga block, and it adjusts to a height that works best for you. Learn more about the Soul Seat on the *Wellness for Makers* podcast.

Stability balls encourage playful movement that helps you build strength in the body by sitting, bending, and wiggling. My stability ball (*pictured*) is by Venn Design. They are beautifully handcrafted by makers in Salem, Oregon. Learn more about Venn Design on the *Wellness for Makers* podcast.

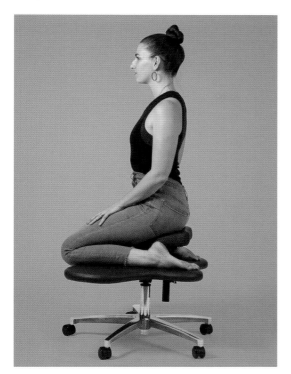

Kneeling

Seated

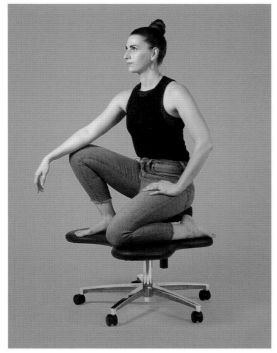

Half squat and half kneeling

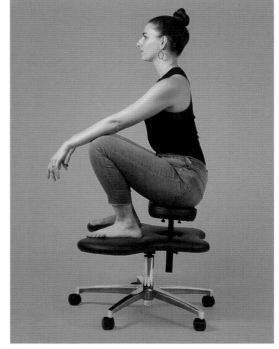

Squatting

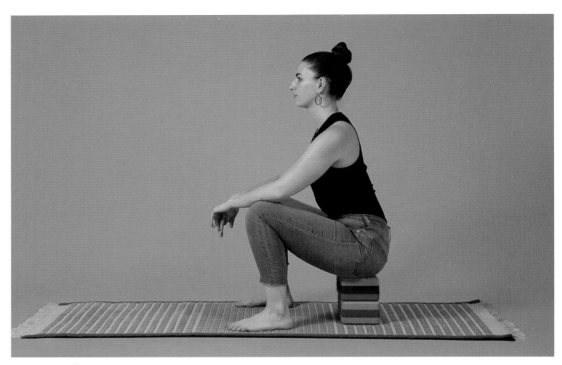

Supported squat

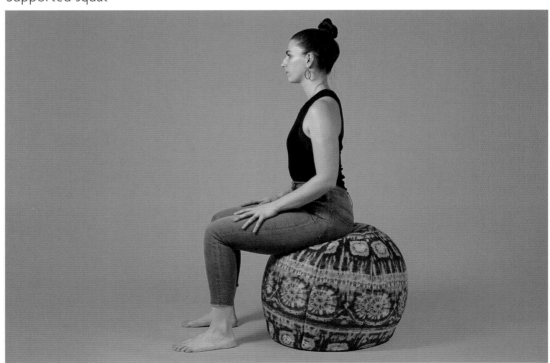

Stability ball

Risk & Repair

Acknowledging the risks of making will encourage you to create modifications where necessary. For example, the way you hold and interact with your tools affects your hands, wrists, and forearms. Do you use power tools for extended periods of time? Electric tools speed up the process of making; however, the high-frequency vibrations can damage the blood vessels and nerves in your hands and forearms over time. If you are a jeweler, this is something to be aware of, especially if you use a flex shaft.

To reduce your risk of injury, limit your exposure to power tools and take breaks regularly. If you are unable to limit the amount of time you work with a specific tool, try to modify it to reduce vibration levels, your grip force, or both. Is it possible to add foam or padding to the tool? Some companies have created custom rubber cushions to provide an added layer of comfort, help reduce the impact of the vibration, and loosen your grip. Look into it, try it out, see what works best for you, and notice how you feel in your body.

Loosening your grip can go a long way with a lot of smaller hand tools as well! You can even try using soft-foam pencil grips, which are often used when kids are learning to hold pencils. You might begin to notice that your hands cramp a little less than when you were clenching your fist to hold a tool. Foam tubing comes in a variety of different thicknesses and can be found at your local hardware store. The goal is to reduce your grip force!

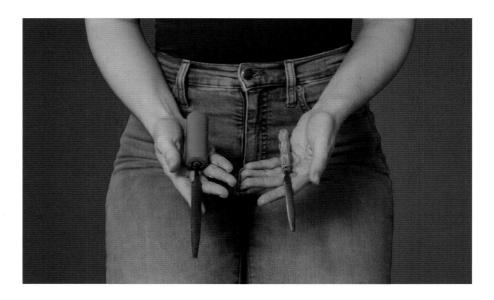

If you lean onto the edge of a table, consider the force you are applying to your forearms and nerves beneath the skin. The ulnar nerve becomes very vulnerable in this type of position. If you begin to notice how the postures you are in often affect the way you feel, you can begin to move in a way that allows your body to mend.

Add padding or foam to the edge of your workbench, your desk, or even the splash pan of your ceramics wheel to reduce the amount of pressure going into your forearms. Whenever you make a modification, remember that it is important to check in to see if you are actually feeling a shift in your body after using it. Did it help, or do you need to revisit the adjustment?

Mirrors can be a great addition to your workspace to remind you to check in with your posture. They can also act as a tool that lets you see a different angle of your piece, depending on what you are working on. I had a great conversation on the *Wellness for Makers* podcast with Stephanie M. Wilhelm, who suggested that ceramic artists use a mirror while they throw on the wheel to see the profile of their piece. I find this to be a great suggestion that can be used across crafts to check in with your alignment while working. Where can you add a mirror to create a new option?

Surfaces & Terrain

Which types of surfaces do you stand on the most (hard wood, concrete, tile, carpet, etc.)? Try alternating from harder floors to an antifatigue mat or textured sensory mat throughout the day. This action will allow you to incorporate some extra variety in your movement patterns, alleviate strain on your joints, improve balance, and increase sensory input. Does your practice allow you to alternate between wearing shoes and working barefoot? If not, "sensory insoles" are a great option for stimulating your feet.

Movement Tracker

Take note of your movement breaks throughout the day. Remember that movement means to change position. Stand up, stretch, walk around, dance, wiggle, and switch tasks often. Trust me, your body will thank you!

MONDAY	TUESDAY
WEDNESDAY	**THURSDAY**
FRIDAY	**SATURDAY**
SUNDAY	**TAKEAWAYS**

Movement Tracker

Take note of your movement breaks throughout the day. Remember that movement means to change position. Stand up, stretch, walk around, dance, wiggle, and switch tasks often. Trust me, your body will thank you!

MONDAY	**TUESDAY**
WEDNESDAY	**THURSDAY**
FRIDAY	**SATURDAY**
SUNDAY	**TAKEAWAYS**

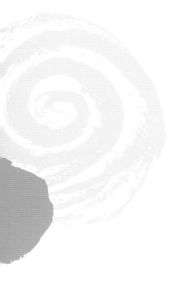

CHAPTER 7 CONSISTENCY

When you learn to move well, your body has the ability to mend itself one thread at a time. Whether you are conscious of it or not, you are always creating either positive or negative change in your body.

It's up to you to decide how you want to engage with that change over time. Is your goal to create a lasting studio practice? If so, keep in mind that building longevity in your movement patterns requires consistent effort.

Practice finding neutral in your postures and movements to develop a stronger connection to your body. Use it as a reference point to understand how your studio movements make you feel. Remember that you don't have to throw out any one movement entirely. The goal is to introduce as much variety as possible. Incorporate more movement breaks with massage, strengthening, and active stretching techniques to alleviate pain and strain. Counterbalance your most common movements, so you can engage with them more mindfully over time.

If your goal is to stand more or move more throughout the day, build up slowly. For example, you don't have to toss all of your chairs to the curb and never sit again. Begin standing for short periods of time more often. This book is an invitation for you to become more aware of your body's movement needs. Incorporate more movement breaks and set reminders to counterbalance your most repetitive movements with stretching, strengthening, and massage techniques.

I hope that at this point you are feeling inspired to incorporate some positive changes into your everyday routine. We often know that we should move, but we end up putting it off. Try leaving yourself reminders to move, stretch, massage, hydrate, and readjust. If you notice yourself beginning to ignore the reminders, find a new way to notify yourself to engage with the practice.

If you've invested in self-care tools and find yourself forgetting to use them because they are tucked away in a drawer, place them purposefully in your space so they cannot be ignored. The more consistent you are about practicing the content of this book, the more you will get out of it. The time you spend creating your art can be an opportunity to get stronger and move more effectively in the studio.

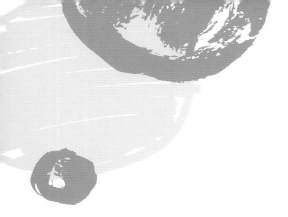

CHAPTER 8 CLOSING NOTE

Hey Maker,

Your dedication to improving your studio practice is inspiring. As you move forward, I challenge you to question the way you have done things in the past and encourage you to make choices that have a positive impact on your body, mind, and studio practice.

Thank you so much for offering me the opportunity to guide you through this process. I invite you to come back to this book again and again to get the most out of the information presented. Remember that there is always more to learn. Even the best teachers are forever students.

This might be the end of this book, but our journey together is just beginning. Inspired to learn more? I have so much to share with you. The Wellness for Makers website is a great place to gain access to videos, products mentioned in this book, courses, and upcoming workshops. Tune into the Wellness for Makers podcast to learn more from a wide range of perspectives.

Ready to transform the content in this book into a consistent movement practice? Visit https://www.wellnessformakers.com to gain access to courses, movement break class packs, and more.

Finally, if you enjoyed the book, I'd love to hear from you! Please share your story with me at info@wellnessformakers.com or connect with me on social media @wellnessformakers.

Keep learning. Keep moving. Keep making.

Xo,

Missy

NOTES

Introduction

1. Thomas Fuller, *Gnomologia: Adagies and Proverbs, Wise Sentences and Witty Sayings, Ancient and Modern, Foreign and British*, collected by Thomas Fuller, MD (Dublin, Ireland: S. Powell, 1733), 283.

Chapter 1: Why We Move

1. Additional information about how movement and lack of movement affect the human body: Katy Bowman, *Move Your DNA* (Sequim, WA: Propriometrics Press, 2017).

2. A quick animated overview of the different ways that sitting affects the human body: Murat Dalkilinç, "Why Sitting Is Bad for You," TED-Ed, March 2015, YouTube video, https://www.ted.com/talks/murat_dalkilinc_why_sitting_is_bad_for_you.

3. Recent research about the benefits of replacing a small amount of sedentary time throughout the day with light or moderate intensity movement: Keith M. Diaz, Andrea T. Duran, Natalie Colabianchi, Suzanne E. Judd, and Virginia J. Howard, "Potential Effects on Mortality of Replacing Sedentary Time with Short Sedentary Bouts or Physical Activity: A National Cohort Study," *American Journal of Epidemiology* 188, no. 3 (March 2019): 537.

4. Bowman, *Move Your DNA*.

Chapter 2: Why We Mend

1. Jules Mitchell, *Yoga Biomechanics: Stretching Redefined* (Pencaitland, Scotland: Handspring, 2019), 176.

Chapter 3: Finding Neutral

1. Additional information about anatomical neutral: Blandine Calais-Germain, *Anatomy of Movement* (Seattle, WA: Eastland, 1985), 7.

2. An overview of proprioception, kinesthesia, and how they work together: "Proprioception and Kinesthesia," Khan Academy, https://www.khanacademy.org/test-prep/mcat/processing-the-environment/somatosensation/v/roprioception-kinesthesia.

3. Emily N. Ussery, Janet E. Fulton, Deborah A. Galuska, Peter T. Katzmarzyk, and Susan A. Carlson, "Joint Prevalence of Sitting Time and Leisure-Time Physical Activity among US Adults, 2015–2016," *JAMA* 320, no. 19 (November 20, 2018): 2036.

4. Diaz et al., "Replacing Sedentary Time," 188.

5. "Take a Deep Breath," *Harvard Mental Health Letter*, May 2009.

6. A visual explanation of how sitting with crossed legs affects your spine: "Legs Crossed?," Ryde Chiropractic, March 12, 2018, https://www.rydechiropractic.com.au/sitting-legs-crossed-bad/.

7. Additional information about foot health and barefoot movement: The Barefoot Movement, https://www.thebarefootmovement.com.au; and Katy Bowman, *Whole Body Barefoot* (Sequim, WA: Propriometrics Press, 2015).

8. Aaron Kucyi, Tim V. Salomons, and Karen D. Davis, "Brain Dynamics of Mind Wandering Away from Pain," *Proceedings of the National Academy of Sciences* 110, no. 46 (November 2013): 18692–97, https://doi.org/10.1073/pnas.1312902110; and Karen D. Davis, "How Does Your Brain Respond to Pain?," TED-Ed, June 2, 2014, YouTube video, https://www.youtube.com/watch?v=I7wfDenj6CQ.

Chapter 4: Studio Movements & Misalignments

1. Michael Rosengart, "List of Common Compensation Patterns and Movement Dysfunctions," Prehab Exercises, https://prehabexercises.com/compensation-patterns/.

2. Mitchell, *Yoga Biomechanics*.

3. Kristian Berg, *Prescriptive Stretching* (Champaign, IL: Human Kinetics, 2011).

4. Carson Demers, *Knitting Comfortably: The Ergonomics of Handknitting* (San Francisco: Ergo I, 2016).

Chapter 5: Mending

1. Fuller, *Gnomologia*.

2. Jean-Claude Guimberteau, *Architecture of Human Living Fascia* (Edinburgh: Handspring, 2016).

3. Thomas Myers, "What Am I Feeling? Recent Research on Interoceptive Sensors of the Myofascia," *Massage Magazine*, December 18, 2018, https://www.massagemag.com/interoceptive-sensors-of-the-myofascia-109064/.

4. Sue Hitzmann, *The Melt Method* (New York: HarperOne, 2013).

5. Mitchell, *Yoga Biomechanics*.

6. Ibid.

BIBLIOGRAPHY

Bengochea, Kim. "Pronation and Supination." Kenhub Anatomy. Last modified October 29, 2020. https://www.kenhub.com/en/library/anatomy/pronation-and-supination.

Berg, Kristian. *Prescriptive Stretching*. Champaign, IL: Human Kinetics, 2011.

Bowman, Katy. *Alignment Matters*. Sequim, WA: Propriometrics Press, 2019.

Bowman, Katy. *Movement Matters*. Sequim, WA: Propriometrics Press, 2016.

Bowman, Katy. *Move Your DNA*. Sequim, WA: Propriometrics Press, 2017.

Bowman, Katy. "Move Your DNA: The Difference between Exercise and Movement (and Why It Matters)." Florida Institute for Human & Machine Cognition, March 5, 2019. YouTube video, 1:10. https://www.youtube.com/watch?v=Ytb3h5vhFX4.

Bowman, Katy. *Whole Body Barefoot*. Sequim, WA: Propriometrics Press, 2015.

Bowman, Katy. "You Don't Know Squat." Nutritious Movement. Last updated February 2020. https://www.nutritiousmovement.com/you-dont-know-squat/.

Calais-Germain, Blandine. *Anatomy of Movement*. Seattle, WA: Eastland, 1985.

Capobianco, Robyn. "Anatomy 101: Are Muscular Engagement Cues Doing More Harm Than Good?" *Yoga Journal*. Last modified July 22, 2018. https://www.yogajournal.com/teach/science-behind-cues-in-yoga-anatomy/.

Capobianco, Robyn, and Jana Montgomery. "Anatomy 101: Can You Safely Jump Back to Plank?" *Yoga Journal*. Last modified April 30, 2018. https://www.yogajournal.com/teach/anatomy-101-can-you-safely-jump-back-to-plank/.

Chaitow, Leon. "Fascial Well-Being: Mechanotransduction in Manual and Movement Therapies." *Journal of Bodywork & Movement Therapies* 22 (2018): 235–36.

Dalkilinç, Murat. "The Benefits of Good Posture." TED-Ed, July 2015. YouTube video. https://www.ted.com/talks/murat_dalkilinc_the_benefits_of_good_posture.

Dalkilinç, Murat. "Why Sitting Is Bad for You." TED-Ed, March 2015. YouTube video. https://www.ted.com/talks/murat_dalkilinc_why_sitting_is_bad_for_you.

Davis, Karen D. "How Does Your Brain Respond to Pain?" TED-Ed, June 2, 2014. YouTube video. https://www.youtube.com/watch?v=I7wfDenj6CQ.

Demers, Carson. *Knitting Comfortably: The Ergonomics of Handknitting*. San Francisco: Ergo I, 2016.

Diaz, Keith M., Andrea T. Duran, Natalie Colabianchi, Suzanne E. Judd, and Virginia J. Howard. "Potential Effects on Mortality of Replacing Sedentary Time with Short Sedentary Bouts or Physical Activity: A National Cohort Study." *American Journal of Epidemiology* 188, no. 3 (March 2019): 537–44. https://doi.org/10.1093/aje/kwy271.

Doto, Bob. *The Power of Stretching*. Beverly, MA: Fair Winds, 2020.

Ellis, Christopher. "Active Stretching vs. Passive Stretching." Dynamic Physiotherapy. Last modified December 5, 2019. https://www.dpt.services/blog/2019/12/5/active-stretching-vs-passive-stretching.

Foster, Ariele. "Fascia Release for Yoga." Aim Health U. Accessed November 20, 2020. https://www.aimhealthyu.com/learn/course/fascia-release-for-yoga/.

Fuller, Thomas. *Gnomologia: Adagies and Proverbs, Wise Sentences and Witty Sayings, Ancient and Modern, Foreign and British*. Collected by Thomas Fuller, MD. Dublin, Ireland: S. Powell, 1733.

Garrison, Liz. "Deep Tissue: What Are Knots, Adhesions, and Trigger Points?" Elements Massage. Last modified December 22, 2014. https://elementsmassage.com/preston-hollow/blog/deep-tissue-what-are-knots-adhesions-and-trigger-points-.

Glick, John P. "Down the Spinal Canal: From Herniation to Rupture." *Studio Potter* 29, no. 1 (2001): 57–60.

Glick, John P. "To Sciatica and Back: A Potter's Journey." *Studio Potter* 15, no. 2 (1987): 27–31.

Graff Ballone, Missy, host. "Get More Out of Your Clay with Stephanie Wilhelm." *Wellness for Makers* (podcast), March 20, 2020. Accessed October 22, 2020. https://podcasts.apple.com/us/podcast/wellness-for-makers/id1499175094?i=1000468944506.

Graff Ballone, Missy, host. "Inner Workout with Taylor Elyse Morrison." *Wellness for Makers* (podcast), June 26, 2020. Accessed January 13, 2020. https://podcasts.apple.com/us/podcast/wellness-for-makers/id1499175094?i=1000479688302.

Graff Ballone, Missy, host. "Neuroscience Meets Art and Design with Amanda Phingbodhipakkiya." *Wellness for Makers* (podcast), August 14, 2020. Accessed January 13, 2021. https://podcasts.apple.com/us/podcast/wellness-for-makers/id1499175094?i=1000488092445.

Graff Ballone, Missy, host. "Pain and Movement with Omni Kitts Ferrara." *Wellness for Makers* (podcast), August 7, 2020. Accessed February 6, 2021. https://podcasts.apple.com/us/podcast/wellness-for-makers/id1499175094?i=1000487414389.

Graff Ballone, Missy, host. "Studio Ergonomics with Carson Demers." *Wellness for Makers* (podcast), April 17, 2020. Accessed October 22, 2020. https://podcasts.apple.com/us/podcast/wellness-for-makers/id1499175094?i=1000471825489.

Graff Ballone, Missy, host. "Which Chair Should I Use? With Pack Matthews." *Wellness for Makers* (podcast), October 5, 2020. Accessed November 12, 2020. https://podcasts.apple.com/us/podcast/wellness-for-makers/id1499175094?i=1000493674672.

Graff Ballone, Missy, host. "Wiggle while You Work with Tyler Benner of Venn Design." *Wellness for Makers* (podcast), February 22, 2021. Accessed February, 2021. https://podcasts.apple.com/us/podcast/wellness-for-makers/id1499175094?i=1000510258733.

Greene, Lauriann, and Richard Goggins. *Save Your Hands!* 2nd ed. Coconut Creek, FL: Body of Work Books, 2008.

Guimberteau, Jean-Claude. *Architecture of Human Living Fascia*. Edinburgh: Handspring, 2016.

Healthcare Triage. "Sitting vs. Standing. Is Your Sedentary Life Killing You?" August 24, 2015. YouTube video. https://www.youtube.com/watch?v=N8tE6zSPJ7w.

Hennen, Tisha. "Forearm Flares." January 20, 2021. YouTube video. https://www.youtube.com/watch?v=rJJVwe-on5k.

Hitzmann, Sue. *The Melt Method*. New York: HarperOne, 2013.

Kieffer, Kristen. "PSA: Standing to Throw & Potter Ergonomics." Kristen Kieffer Ceramics, 2016. https://kiefferceramics.com/2018/01/01/psa-standing-ergonomics/.

Kim, Alina. *Kinesiology Taping for Rehab and Injury Prevention*. Berkeley, CA: Ulysses, 2016.

"Kinesthetic Awareness and Proprioception." Core Walking. Accessed January 8, 2021. https://corewalking.com/kinesthetic-awareness-proprioception/.

Kitts-Ferrara, Omni. "Work Better: Yoga Mechanics." Vimeo video. Accessed February 3, 2021. https://vimeo.com/364884907/d9b86bc56a.

Kucyi, Aaron, Tim V. Salomons, and Karen D. Davis. "Brain Dynamics of Mind Wandering Away from Pain." *Proceedings of the National Academy of Sciences* 110, no. 46 (November 2013): 18692–97. https://doi.org/10.1073/pnas.1312902110.

"Legs Crossed?" Ryde Chiropractic. March 12, 2018. https://www.rydechiropractic.com.au/sitting-legs-crossed-bad/.

Matthews, Pack. TEDxCoMo, April 22, 2013. YouTube video. https://www.youtube.com/watch?v=M2NHvpM9PWU.

Mauro, Charles L., Emily Fisher, David Korpan, and P. Adrian Medrano. "Ergonomic Redesign of a Traditional Jewelry-Polishing Workstation." *Ergonomics in Design: The Quarterly of Human Factors Applications* 23, no. 1 (January 2015): 4–12.

McCreight, Tim. *Complete Metalsmith*. Portland, ME: Brynmorgen, 2004.

Miller, Jill. *The Roll Model*. Las Vegas, NV: Victory Belt, 2014.

Mitchell, Jules. "Loading and Stretching." Yoga Biomechanics. Last modified June 26, 2016. https://www.julesmitchell.com/loading-and-stretching/.

Mitchell, Jules. *Yoga Biomechanics: Stretching Redefined*. Pencaitland, Scotland: Handspring, 2019.

"Muscle Pain: It May Actually Be Your Fascia." Johns Hopkins Medical. Accessed January 27, 2021. https://www.hopkinsmedicine.org/health/wellness-and-prevention/muscle-pain-it-may-actually-be-your-fascia.

Myers, Tom. "Fascia 101." Functional Patterns, November 20, 2014. YouTube video. https://www.youtube.com/watch?v=-uzQMn87Hg0.

Myers, Tom. "What Am I Feeling? Recent Research on Interoceptive Sensors of the Myofascia." *Massage Magazine*, December 18, 2018. https://www.massagemag.com/interoceptive-sensors-of-the-myofascia-109064/.

Myers, Tom. "What You Need to Know about Fascia." *Yoga Journal*. Last modified January 18, 2018. https://www.yogajournal.com/teach/anatomy-yoga-practice/what-you-need-to-know-about-fascia-2/.

Naboso. "Benefits of Barefoot Stimulation for Children." *Naboso* (blog), August 23, 2019. https://www.naboso.com/blogs/the-bare-foot-advantage/benefits-of-barefoot-stimulation-for-children.

Nestor, James. *Breath: The New Science of a Lost Art*. New York: Riverhead Books, 2020.

Phingbodhipakkiya, Amanda. "How Design Can Help Make Science Accessible." TED Archive, April 23, 2018. YouTube video. https://www.youtube.com/watch?v=FvI_cseAVeU.

Phingbodhipakkiya, Amanda. "The Storytelling of Science." TED Residency, November 21, 2016. YouTube video. https://www.youtube.com/watch?v=HC5theZw3FE.

Piegorsch, Karen. "An Ergonomic Bench for Indigenous Weavers." Human Factors and Ergonomics Society, 2009.

"Proprioception and Kinesthesia." Khan Academy. Accessed December 19, 2020. https://www.khanacademy.org/test-prep/mcat/processing-the-environment/somatosensation/v/proprioception-kinesthesia.

Rodabaugh, Katrina. *Mending Matters*. New York: Abrams, 2018.

Rosengart, Michael. "List of Common Compensation Patterns and Movement Dysfunctions." Prehab Exercises. Accessed November 15, 2020. https://prehabexercises.com/compensation-patterns/.

Slon, Stephanie, and Julie Corliss. *Healthy Hands: Strategies, for Strong, Pain-Free Hands*. Special Health Report from Harvard Medical School. Boston: Harvard Health, 2015.

Suzuki, Wendy. "The Brain-Changing Benefits of Exercise." TEDWomen 2017, November 2017. TED video. https://www.ted.com/talks/wendy_suzuki_the_brain_changing_benefits_of_exercise.

"Take a Deep Breath." *Harvard Mental Health Letter*, May 2009.

"The Truth about Standing Desks." Med School Insiders, December 15, 2018. YouTube video. https://www.youtube.com/watch?v=yhkigA368mE.

Ussery, Emily N., Janet E. Fulton, Deborah A. Galuska, Peter T. Katzmarzyk, and Susan A. Carlson. "Joint Prevalence of Sitting Time and Leisure-Time Physical Activity among US Adults, 2015–2016." *JAMA* 320, no. 19 (November 20, 2018): 2036–38. https://doi.org/10.1001/jama.2018.17797.

Vagy, Jared. "Warm-up Right: How to Prep Wrists and Fingers to Send." *Climbing Magazine*. Last modified August 21, 2018. https://www.climbing.com/skills/warm-up-right-how-to-prep-wrists-and-fingers-to-send/.

Wilhelm, Stephanie M. "Educational Resources." Accessed February 16, 2021. https://www.stephaniemwilhelm.com/educational-resources.html.

Wilson, Jean. "Ergonomics for Jewelry Makers." *Art Jewelry Magazine*, 2010.

ACKNOWLEDGMENTS

I am so grateful for the opportunity to write this book, share strategies and techniques that have changed my life, and shift the perspective of movement in the artist studio. Thank you to the amazing team at Schiffer Publishing, in particular Sandra Korinchak, senior editor, for reaching out to create this book. Thank you for believing in the importance of this topic and bringing it to the rest of the team. To Karla Rosenbusch, senior editor, for editing the book and engaging with the material. I appreciate all of your excitement and patience as we brought the book to life!

To Angelique Hanesworth, of Eye Spy Photography, for spending countless hours photographing and editing all of the amazing images in the book. Thank you for encouraging me throughout the process so I could make sure that all the photos were in the position or alignment I needed for the explanations in the book. To Julianna Brazill for being a huge part of the Wellness for Makers brand since the beginning. Thank you for every illustration you've created throughout the years and for always helping make my vision come to life. To everyone that I have interviewed through the *Wellness for Makers* podcast. Thank you for sharing your work, stories, and perspectives. You have helped solidify my thoughts and shape my perspective. You are each evidence of the power and importance of community.

To my husband, Jonathan, for sharing an interest in movement with me. Thank you for all of the late nights that you joined me in proofreading and researching without hesitation. I am forever grateful for your love, support, and commitment. To my incredible mother for answering the phone multiple times a day. Thank you for continuing to cheer me on and offering me ongoing love and support. To my dearest friends who stood by me, offered honest feedback, and cheered me on throughout the process. Thank you for being you!

To my network of family, friends, and colleagues who have supported me in this work since the beginning. Though there are too many to name, your encouragement means the world to me. To all of my art teachers who have helped me grow and establish my creative career. Thank you for every opportunity and every letter of recommendation, and for teaching me to think critically about the way I structure and brand my work. To all of my movement instructors for teaching me how to move more effectively in my own life. Thank you for believing that the best teachers in life are forever students first. I am excited to see what I learn next!

Thank you to my incredible students, readers, and online community. Your excitement and encouragement give me the confidence to continue this important work. To all the schools, shops, galleries, and studios who plan to carry and promote this book. Thank you for spreading the word and sharing your ongoing support as we shift the perspective of what it means to move well in the studio. All of you mean the world to me.

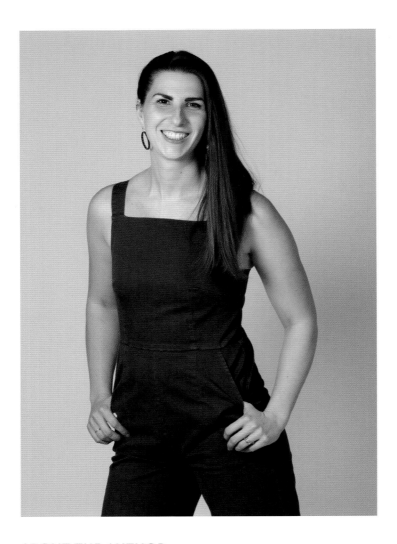

ABOUT THE AUTHOR

Missy Graff Ballone is an artist, licensed massage therapist, yoga instructor RYT 500, and movement educator. She created Wellness for Makers® to provide artists and craftsmen with accessible, relevant, and empowering wellness resources. Missy draws from her extensive training and continuing education to find new ways to inspire creatives to move well in the studio. She also hosts the Wellness for Makers podcast and interviews artists and movement professionals from around the world. Missy lives and creates in Hudson Valley, New York.